My Roller Coaster Ride
With

GOD
and
CANCER

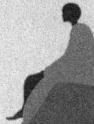

Then, Sitting With Him On the Brink of Eternity

Gordon Ferguson

Cover design by Roy Appalsamy. Layout by Toney C. Mulhollan.

Theatron Press cares deeply for the environment and uses recycled papers whenever possible.

ISBN: 978-1-958723-31-9.

About the author: Gordon Ferguson is a graduate of Northwestern State University and the Harding School of Theology. With more than fifty years of experience, he has served as an evangelist, elder and teacher. Gordon has written nineteen books and produced many audio/video teaching series. He and his wife, Theresa, have two adult children and five grandchildren and live in McKinney, Texas. For additional information about his work and ministry go to www.GordonFerguson.org.

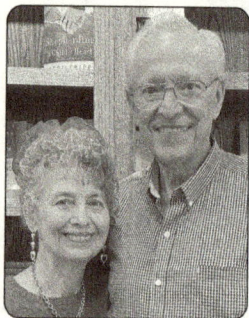

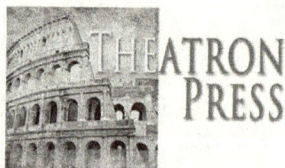

THEATRON
PRESS

Theatron Press is an imprint of Illumination Publishers International
www.ipibooks.com

Dedication

To All Those Affected by Cancer

Most of the dedication pages I have written for my books have been totally positive in tone. This one is different but no less heartfelt, in fact probably moreso. Everyone reading this book has been affected by cancer. Some of you are fighting your personal battle with it right now or have a close loved one who is. Others of you have lost loved ones who were unable to win their battle with this dreaded disease. Some of you are like me, cancer survivors, but we will always live with the thought that it might return.

I keep a long prayer list of people who seriously need prayers for a variety of reasons. One part of the list contains the names of those currently fighting cancer. That section has twenty-five names on it. One passed recently and I removed his name, but then put his wife's name (and family) on the list of ones grieving the loss of those dearest to them. Every day as I pray, I am reminded of those and their families who are where I was in 2022 during my battle, which is described in this book.

I wrote the book to encourage you, regardless of how you may be affected by cancer when you are reading it. I am gut-level honest about my wide emotional swings and the challenges I felt during my wild ride, the worst of which was due to the treatment and not the cancer itself, an unusual circumstance. I hope to mostly encourage you with my encounters with God during my ride and the results it produced in my life. Like many have said before me, as rough as the ride was, I would not remove that chapter of my life if I could. I needed it and I will need the lessons I learned from it when my time to meet God does come. At 82 years of age, it can't be too far away. But until that day comes, I have today, the same as everyone else, and I am going to live it to the full. Please join me in that, and may God bless you!

Contents

Contents

Introduction

CANCER. That's a really scary word to most people. I remember being with my dad when the doctor told him he had cancer. Hearing it almost took my breath away. Daddy and I had become very close friends in my adult years. He lived another six years, but that word always hung in the air when I was with him. It was a tough six years for him and for those who watched him endure treatments and surgeries. In June of 2021, I had my third rectal surgery. The pathology reports began as indecisive but later progressed to a diagnosis of adenocarcinoma. "Mr. Ferguson, you have cancer."

At the initial *indecisive* stage, the surgeon said that she needed to go back in and get a deeper sample, and she would get the best margins she could in an attempt to get all of the cancer if it were cancer. Oddly perhaps, hearing that wasn't scary to me at the time. I simply told the doctor that we all have a shelf life, and I was almost 79 at the time and had lived a very blessed life. As I have aged, I often think of the old version of Psalm 90:10, "The days of our years are threescore years and ten; and if by reason of strength they be fourscore years, yet is their strength labour and sorrow; for it is soon cut off, and we fly away." I couldn't help but wonder if I would "fly away" in my 80th year.

After that surgery ten days later, the pathology report came back clear. She wanted to see me again every few months to remove tissue in her office for continuing tests. It was after the second of those on December 29th that led to the call on January 5, 2022, saying that I did have adenocarcinoma and would need to set up treatments right away with oncologists. She seemed positive about radiation being able to cure it and promised to have an oncology service contact me for an appointment. At that point, I was amazingly calm and at peace. Surrendered. I slept like a baby that night. The first item on my prayer list about my condition was to not have cancer, but if I did, that it would be God's way of exposing it early so it could be treated successfully.

The second item on that prayer list started with the words, "More importantly," followed by a request that no matter what happened with the cancer, up to and including a terminal stage of it, that I would trust God and his timing implicitly and un-questionably. So, in any case, my prayers were being answered and I was at peace, a truly wonderful feeling, that peace that surpasses human understanding as described in Philippians 4:7. This was the beginning of my journey, my roller coaster ride with God and cancer. Before it was done, I would be led to the very edge of death, not knowing if I would live or die. At that stage, I pictured myself sitting on the brink of eternity with God. The physical experience was horrific, but the spiritual experience was euphoric. That combination prompted the insights found in Part Two of this book.

The Prayers of Spiritual Friends

After I received my diagnosis of cancer, I posted a request for prayers on my Facebook page to my 5,000 FB friends. For years, I have prayed through a long prayer list kept on my computer, asking God to bless specific people with all kinds of needs, some of whom I didn't know personally, along with their families and all who were impacted by their situation. I believe that simply the mention of their names and problems to God makes a difference. On the days when doing this seems a bit laborious, after having finished my prayer times about personal matters, I always had this thought: one day I am go-ing to be in a serious situation in which I am going to want my name brought before God's throne by as many as possible.

With that motivation, I nearly always get past my selfishness and respond to the Golden Rule of Jesus and pray through my ever-growing list.

That "one day" for me became Wednesday, January 5, 2022. The response to my request was overwhelming. I can't stop crying right now as I write this. God has been kind beyond comprehension in giving me so many friends. At my age, most of them are as my spiritual children. They care deeply and want to help, just like my physical son and his family. Our son, Bryan, and his wife, Joy, asked us to move close to them, for two reasons. One, to enjoy their three sons while they were still just kids, since they had lived in Hawaii for 25 years and the boys were fast approaching adulthood. When we moved to Dallas at the end of 2014, a mile from where they now live, Bryce (Bryce Gordon, by the way) was in high school, Blayze was in middle school and Ronan was in elementary school. Watching them grow into men has been indeed special.

Two, they wanted to help take care of us as age takes its toll on us, which it inevitably does. They both have the hearts of natural caretakers. In his mature years, Bryan went back to school to obtain a master's degree in counseling. Joy, as a nurse, truly has the heart of a servant. Although we haven't yet needed much help from them, they still look for opportunities to give it. We are ever so thankful that our son and daughter by marriage (daughter-in-law doesn't work for us) wanted us to live close by. It has been a very special chapter in our lives. God has seen fit to bless us with many who share that same heart for us, and it is very humbling and wonderful beyond words. The scope of our blessings far surpasses anything we deserve, especially me, which speaks volumes about God and the impact of Jesus upon the lives of those whom he has brought into our lives.

Into a Writer's Mind

I do a lot of prayer journaling. As a writer, I can express my feelings better through typing than through speaking or writing with pen and paper. On most days, I don't save what I write. It is very personal and not something I would want others to read, for a number of reasons. You can understand that I imagine. Because of the wild emotional and spiritual roller coaster ride that started on January 5th, with its unexpected twists and turns, I knew instinctively that I needed to save what I wrote. In this case, I wanted to keep a record of the events and my prayers in response to those events. I thought of possible book titles in the process, in which to include what I was writing as a framework for them at some future point. The title of this book was not among them, for I had not yet looked at death in the face over a prolonged period.

I wrote and saved my writing early in my cancer journey because I felt compelled to record what God was doing in my life, the insights I was gaining and the spiritual growth I was experiencing. I was unburdening my heart and having my heart filled by God at the very same time. As will be obvious, I am an emotionally based person, and despite the fact that describing my wide-ranging emotions is a bit embarrassing, openness and vulnerability is an essential part of facing serious health challenges. From the earliest days, it has been a life-changing journey. On February 7th, which happened to fall on the 19th birthday of our fourth grandson, Cody, who lives in Arizona, I received the results of two scans and a key blood test. No cancer. (A mistaken diagnosis, as we will see.)

As I mentioned in a FB post a day later, that report put me in shock. I did have the faith as I prayed beforehand that it was not only possible that God might heal me, but probable. Prayers offered by so many people all over the world simply had to make a difference. That said, it was still a shock.

After sharing the details with Theresa about it all, putting her in shock with me, I went on a long prayer walk. At one point along the way, and I remember exactly where I was at the time, a thought hit me that caused me to burst into tears. It was not produced by a sense of relief that I didn't have cancer, although I was understandably very, very relieved. It wasn't caused by a heightened feeling of gratitude, although I was filled with gratitude.

That overwhelming thought was the realization of how much the past month had changed me spiritually. I told God that I would not eliminate a single thing in that wild and scary ride or change it in any way. I told him that I would rather have the cancer back than lose what I had gained spiritually. And I meant every word of it. I still mean it. Being in my 81st year of life means that I am nearing my end anyway. When that comes, I won't feel any differently than I do now about life and death. The real me, the part made in God's image, doesn't age. Only the body ages and passes away. Plus, time goes by fast. I will be on death's door soon enough. Staying alive on planet earth isn't the big issue or anywhere close to it. Staying close to God and falling more and more in love with him is the big issue. Actually, it's about the only issue. Now let's board the coaster and let the ride begin. Front row, please, where the thrills are the most intense.

PART ONE
The Roller Coaster Ride

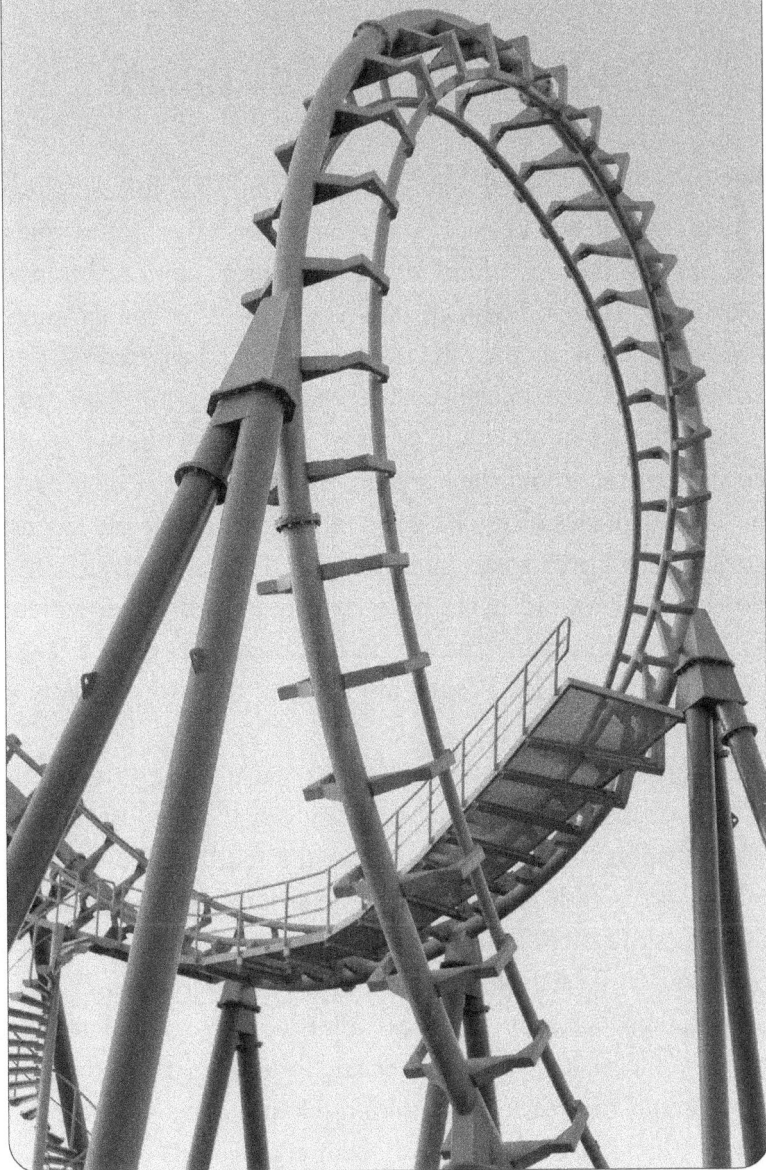

Chapter 1

•

Pulling Out of the Station

I am a roller coaster buff and an adrenaline junkie. I love adventure. My childhood was filled with thrills and spills as a result of my often unwise and unsafe choices, but my, was it fun! The God who created us knows us intimately and I believe he fashions the directions our lives take based on this knowledge of what makes us tick. That has certainly been true in my life. The number and types of adventures I have experienced and totally relished are simply amazing as I look back on the memories of my 81 years of life. But as the old saying goes, into all lives some rain must fall. I have survived some downpours I would never have chosen, adventures complete with those adrenaline rushes, but endured with gritted teeth and an aching heart. What I am describing in this book is a combination of both types.

Like all roller coaster rides, the early stage is exciting as the ascent begins, but it is mostly just the anticipation of what is soon to come. Then comes the first big drop, which takes your breath away. My initial peace following my initial diagnosis of cancer lasted just over twenty-four hours and was beautiful while it lasted. However, that was soon to change and change radically. The next afternoon, I decided to call Mark Mancini, a fellow minister and longtime friend, to learn more about the effects of radiation. He did cover that, for his surgery had failed to remove all the margins of his cancer, thus necessitating radiation treatment. His situation reminded me of my father's surgery that ultimately led to his death, a result of the surgeon not removing all of the margins, leaving cancer where it shouldn't have been. I couldn't help wondering if that might be true in my own case as well, an unsettling thought.

But back to the unexpected direction in my conversation with Mark. His main emphasis was his absolute insistence that I contact the University of Texas Southwestern Medical Center for a second opinion. To say that he was pushy would be to make an understatement. He wouldn't let up on that one, which left me very disturbed at the end of the call. I felt like I got robbed of my surrendered sense of peace. I was very troubled and unsettled. I was actually ticked off at Mark, a dear friend. I had never seen him in that pushy mode before.

The question that came to mind at this point is the one that has come up hundreds of times when circumstances seem difficult or impossible to interpret. Was this just another test of my surrender, since I was definitely surrendered prior to the call, or was this a circumstance designed by God to lead me in another direction for treatment? I believe God has sent both my way hundreds of times. I hate the feeling that my wisdom, human wisdom, is in the driver's seat and it's up to me to make the right choices in serious situations. I just despise the idea, a popular one with many people (especially the driven, successful types), that "If it is to be, it is up to me." No, no, no—not that! I want it to be, "If it is to be, it must be up to Thee." But there I was, caught between two choices in interpreting the talk with Mark – a test of surrender or a circumstance designed to lead me in another direction, a needed one. Oh no! Not again!

The Wrestling Match Continues

Like Jacob of old (Genesis 32), I was wrestling with God, but not fully realizing it yet. For the next several days, I was up and down and all around emotionally. Fortunately, those days were very busy ones, occupying my mind (mostly) with other things. Theresa had two doctor's appointments the next day and I had to prepare a lesson to deliver via Zoom the next day, Saturday, for a conference in London. Those events were helpful just as distractions if nothing else.

I watched lots of football that weekend, an NFL playoff weekend, providing more distraction for which I was grateful. But underneath the surface, I remained filled with angst. On Tuesday morning, I had a virtual computer appointment with the oncology radiologist, which generally went well. The proposed treatment sounded about like I expected, and the doctor seemed nice enough and competent enough, answering all my questions well. There was just a hint of arrogance on his part when I mentioned the possibility of getting a second opinion, which made me a bit nervous (God opposes the proud – James 4:6). Otherwise, it was good.

I think it may have been the next morning that I woke up with the memory of what a cheerful, petite redheaded doctor had said in reply to a question I asked her years ago after she had just performed a sigmoidoscopy on me. My curiosity about what would motivate a doctor to pursue a specialty in dealing with this part of the body led me to ask, "Why would a doctor go into this line of work?" A few years earlier, I had asked this same question to another doctor in a similar circumstance, also a female physician, and it flustered her. She just said, "That's a good question" and left the room (and didn't come back).

The little redhead, whose husband was the head of that department, wasn't flustered in the least. "Easy answer," said she. "If you catch this kind of cancer early, you get it every time!" Out of the clear blue that memory appeared. I thought of John 14:26 where Jesus promised the apostles that the Holy Spirit would bring things to their remembrance. I know that this was a promise to them of the Spirit doing it in a miraculously inspired sense, but I have long believed that miraculous gifts of the Spirit have non-miraculous counterparts. So, in my mind, I believed I had been given such a blessing that early morning to ease my mind. It was a special beginning to the day, a needed one.

That Fateful Thursday

On Wednesday, one week after my talk with Mark, I called Mike Isenberg, my friend in church who is a physician assistant. He listened carefully and said that continuity with my present doctors was important if I trusted them and that he thought either place could do the needed job. He did say that UT Southwestern was a great place, but that he didn't think I could make a wrong decision either way. In other words, both would be competent to provide adequate treatment. That was reassuring, as Mike always is, and tilted me back toward feeling good about staying the original course. I even told my sister on the phone that I was almost certainly going to do that and quit being torn between the two options. I felt much more settled out. The only question in the back of my mind was prompted by some underlying feelings about my surgeon. While I liked her and mostly trusted her, I had some lingering doubts in the back of my mind due to some inconsistencies in how she had explained some of the earlier pathology reports. However, I was pretty much settled out about my present reasonably firm decision, yet still a little ticked off at Mark's pushiness.

Since the next day was a nice one outside and I hadn't walked for a while due to the residual pain after my last tissue removal for pathology, I decided to take a walk. I was mostly healed by then, thankfully. As I walked out of the house, I saw my neighbors pull into their driveway and start getting out of their car. We had a little cottage in East Texas at the time (now sold) across the street from a lake and they live directly on the lake. Robin isn't out in the front yard nearly as often as her husband, Harry, but knowing that she had been through cancer treatment recently, I wanted to show her a calm, faithful reaction to having cancer to encourage her. So, we talked. I found out that she had both radiation and chemo for her cancer. Then I had to ask, "Where did you get your treatment?" Of course, it was UT Southwestern—of course it was! And like Mark, she gushed about doing research and UT Southwestern being the best of the best. She wasn't as pushy as Mark, but just as gushy. Okay, unsettledness again. Ugh! The big question popped into my mind once more: test of surrender or circumstantial guidance of the Holy Spirit? Aaaggghhh!!!

Then I continued my walk. Danny and Jynae, neighbors opposite our garage, were out in their yard talking over some construction plans they had for their house. I'd probably not said ten words to Jynae before, and her being out in the front yard was rare. Those on the lake usually hang out in their back yards for obvious reasons, but there they both were. They asked how I was doing, and in my reply, I included the cancer diagnosis and upcoming treatment. Danny said that they had a good friend who just finished with that type of treatment. Keep in mind that I'm talking to people out in the countryside nearly 100 miles from that medical center.

Where their friend lived, I had no idea. They could have lived anywhere in the world. But of course I had to ask the question, right? Of course. When I did, Jynae answered, since it was her female friend who had been treated. By now you can easily guess the answer. UT Southwestern, followed by more glowing reports of this place being the cat's meow, with people coming from all over to go there for cancer treatment. Amazing, simply amazing! What were the odds of this being mere circumstance—both women being out in their front yards on the same day at the same time—in the winter at that? I'd never seen it before. With both women having the same story about UT Southwestern too?

I See You Now, God

Okay, give-up time, God. I'll seriously start looking into the option of getting a second opinion. I began calling that afternoon, but it wasn't a good initial experience. I pushed my #1 phone key at two different times, the option for new patients, and the woman who answered sounded muffled and not nearly on top of her game. Disappointing. Nothing like Mark and Robin had described. I was in a bad place emotionally, to put it mildly, although I didn't show it to avoid unsettling my dear wife. I didn't sleep well that night and felt drained when I awoke the next morning. I had another virtual appointment, with the chemo oncologist this time. She was very pleasant and explained things well and answered my questions thoroughly. But the amount of chemo she described was disturbing. The one positive thing that the call did accomplish was that I was even more motivated to get a second opinion. I did not like the sound of the treatment described and now definitely wanted that second opinion.

That same morning as we started heading back to Dallas for Theresa's two medical appointments, I called UT Southwestern once more, pushing the #1 button for new patients. The same woman answered and still sounded muffled, so I pulled off the road to try understanding what she was saying. It was frustrating and I got nowhere. Not good. I dropped Theresa off at the medical facility for her appointment and tried to take a nap in the car, but I was too geared up to sleep. I called UT Southwestern again, either in the parking lot or right after arriving home, intending to apologize for being a pest but just wanting to see if I had done all I could to move the process forward. I simply could not get through.

The woman or the system finally just hung up on me after a long hold. Aaaggghhh! Again! But by then I was determined to try once more, and this time I pushed the #2 button for "existing patients." When a woman answered, whose name I found out to be Rosie, I explained that I wasn't an existing patient but was trying hard to become one and was hitting roadblocks. She was the type of person Mark and Robin had described – precisely. She was extremely nice and super helpful. I had the thought that she might be an angel. Seriously. She was that good. From there we got the balls rolling in several directions.

She quickly said that she knew exactly which doctor I should see and if everything fell into place, she might be able to schedule me on Wednesday (five days later). Timing meant a lot to me. If cancer metastasizes, it has to begin at a certain point in time, right? That seemed logical. Ahh! Good news, finally. After finding out the referrals and reports they required, I started doing my part. It was Friday afternoon, and their admitting department was about to close for a long weekend, since MLK Day fell on that Monday. But Rosie assured me that if I could get everything in by early Tuesday morning, she would make it happen for that Wednesday appointment. Getting in to see specialists just doesn't happen that way, and I speak from experience. It was almost too good to be true and thus difficult to trust what I had been told.

However, I was set on doing my part as best I could. They wanted reports and referrals from both my surgeon and my primary care physician. I sent written messages through the internet portals of both. I made phone calls and left voicemails, including one to the nurse of my primary care doctor and another to their remote emergency nurse. Then I thought of pushing the button for contacts from doctors or hospitals. When a live person answered that line, I told her that I was calling on behalf of the Simmons Cancer Center at UT Southwestern (*sorta* true). I explained what was going on and she said she would send the needed documentation, hopefully that same afternoon (late Friday afternoon).

The pieces all seem to be falling into place, good places. So far so good, although gut-wrenching at times. Just about then, it hit me that the answer to my question of whether the situation was surrender being tested or the Spirit leading me in another direction was both/and, not either/or. I looked up and said, "Good one, Lord. I hope you are enjoying this. I'm starting to. You are doing your thing again, jumping out from behind bushes to scare the liver out of me. Okay. I've still got a sense of humor and an appreciation of yours. We're good for now. More to come, I'm sure." I often talk to God, not just pray to him. Friends do that, right? (John 15:15)

Where is the Peace?

I was at that point thinking about what was keeping me from being surrendered and at peace again. God knows how much I love being there when I do get there. It is the greatest feeling on his green earth—an at-oneness with him that has no superiors. But I hadn't had it recently, although by that Saturday, I got back close to it. I think my problem was that until I got the UT Southwestern appointment nailed down completely, I couldn't relax enough to be totally at peace. That realization disturbed me. Complete trust in a God who works everything together for good (Romans 8:28) should have produced peace in me. I'm slow to learn, no questioning that, thus slow to trust.

When will I ever learn that God will take care of the details if I will simply just let go and let God? Ferguson, you wrote a book about the victory in surrender.[i] Why in the name of common sense don't you listen to your better self? Goodness gracious! Trust is the issue. The call to Mark set me on my ear. But then the sequence afterwards should have put me in a good place, right? I made out a list of what God had done since that fateful call to Mark, a list of what should have stopped me from being untrusting and stupid. What's the matter with you anyway, Gordon? Why don't you stop this faithless stuff and quit going down rabbit holes? (Do you talk to yourself too?)

Without the absolute pushiness of Mark, I wouldn't have followed through. I needed to hear from Robin and Jynae too, but I wouldn't have reached out to them without Mark's getting under my skin. To top it off, Joy informed me that our mutual friend, Bethany Smith, received her treatment at UT Southwestern too, which was confirmed by her husband Adam. He said a cancer specialist friend in another city advised them to always go to a place connected with a medical school—there you will find the latest and greatest doctors and procedures. I didn't know that Joy even knew Bethany, much less about her cancer treatment. I didn't know about it beforehand myself. That was just one more layer on the cake God was baking.

What else could God possibly have done? Was it easy to get to a surrendered faith? No, but when is it ever with matters that really count? It shouldn't be. It should be a journey of faith, and at times a challenging journey. God is a tester of faith because he is a *builder* of faith. Those two go together. They are actually inseparable. That realization led me to this prayer: "Thanks for persevering with me and revealing yourself to me, Lord. I wish I could see your hand faster with the eye of faith, but just so I end up seeing it, I'm good. And most appreciative. Hold on to me, Father. I'm a mess. But you are the God of unlimited patience who understands messes and loves us anyway. Thank you!"

On Tuesday morning, I awoke on pins and needles once again. On my knees, I asked God's forgiveness and strength to surrender again. After all that had fallen into place by God's providence, why was I not at peace? I determined to call UT

Southwestern at 9:30 am just to make sure they hadn't forgotten me and that the process hadn't been somehow sidetracked. Rosie had promised to call me Tuesday morning. I at least decided to show minimal patience by waiting until 9:30 to call and tried to carry on with my normal morning routine. But I was not at peace. At 9:27 am, I needed to relieve my bladder, and as I was doing so to help three more minutes pass, the phone rang. The caller ID told the story. It was Rosie—my personal angel assigned to me by God. She said she had been working on my case since 8:00 am and I was scheduled for an appointment the very next day.

That was an amazing morning. Surely it would all be downhill from there, right? *Wrong!* My roller coaster rides with God are never short and are always a combination of sheer terror and absolute exhilaration, as roller coaster rides should be. That's why we buy the tickets in the first place, and whether we realized it or not at the time, confessing Jesus as Lord was our request for a ticket to ride and a guarantee that we would receive it. That being true, I (and you) need to stop complaining when it feels like we are coming off the tracks of this thing called life with God and just keep holding on for dear life. Periodic wild rides are part and parcel of what we signed up for in the first place as Christ followers.

Chapter 2

•

The Unexpected Twists and Turns

The first big drop on a roller coaster is a thrill for sure, but it is soon followed by unexpected twists and turns, many of them bone-jarring. Almost all of the coasters I have ridden are very similar in having that initial drop, but from that point forward, usually dissimilar and unpredictable. My ride with God and cancer fit this description all too well. It began with a surreal doctor visit exactly two weeks after receiving my initial cancer diagnosis. When I entered the examination room on that Wednesday, five days from my first contact with Rosie, the nurse came in first and did her thing. Then a resident doctor being trained in this specialty came in and we started talking. He was from Phoenix, where we had lived for nine years, and it turned out we had much in common. We had played many of the same golf courses in Phoenix, for one thing. I mentioned in our conversation that we had lived for sixteen years in Boston prior to moving to Phoenix. As he left the room, I told him it was really good to meet someone from where I had once lived, and he replied, "You will like the doctor then, she is from Boston." Then entered that very impressive specialist from Boston, a Harvard Medical School graduate and a professor at the UT Southwestern Medical School, the largest medical school in Texas.

Her introductory question still gives me chills thinking back on it. *How did you get here?* I deduced from the question that new patients didn't normally start with her. The right answer was God, of course, but working through lots of people and situations, not the least of which was Rosie. When I mentioned Rosie, the doctor laughed, realizing how I got there (from a human perspective). She knew Rosie well it seems. Just amazing, the whole sequence. God didn't violate my free will —but almost. To say he influenced it or even strongly influenced it doesn't quite do justice to what he actually did. Simply mind-boggling amazing! Wow, just wow! I knew it might not work out as well as I hoped. I also knew that one day the other shoe must fall. It is appointed unto all humans once to die, according to Hebrews 9:27, and I wouldn't have it any other way, because that fact of life (and death) is all wrapped up in the greatest story ever told, a story that no one could possibly invent nor even believe at the deepest level. It is too good to be true; too spectacular to be true. But by the eye of faith, we can know it is true anyway—the Creator dying for the created.

So when my end does come, it will be okay. But as another good doctor said in talking about our inevitable death (my old friend, Mark Ottenweller), "I know I am going to die – just not today!" *Yea!* Today I am alive and well and relieved and most grateful to the only One in the universe who deserves all the gratitude received and a googol more. Thank you, Abba! You outdid yourself on this one. Spectacular, and all of the other words that can try and fail to describe you and what you did that day. Praise your holy Name, the Name that is above every name, in heaven and on earth and under the earth. AMEN!

Prayer of January 20—Wonderful Insights!

The thought hit me this night when Theresa came by my office door that she was the greatest miracle of all, that little angel God made especially for me and then made sure I got her. I began thinking about the millions upon millions of miracles that had to occur to make this most important of all human miracles occur, and it is totally mind-boggling. For God just to have put my mother and father together seems impossible—a church girl and a party boy and barroom brawler when they married. I hope to one day find out how they actually got together. I'm sure the details must be quite interesting. But anyway, the miracle of my little angel with whom I had recently celebrated our 57th wedding anniversary is the greatest miracle of all on the human side of life. Thank you, thank you, thank you—I'm beyond words again.

Another insight was about God, me, and our relationship. 2021 was a tough year in some ways, but it was a great year for spiritual growth, needed growth, much needed growth, essential growth. God has given me so much evidence that he was guiding my life in all of its paths that it seems criminal to keep questioning whether he was going to do it "this" time (the current time at any point along life's pathways). Then the thought that hit me is that my definition of surrender focuses on his Lordship in a way different from a Father/son relationship, a love relationship. My early religious background seriously damaged my view of God, and it has taken a long time, too long, to dismantle it and replace it with a more biblical view. I just want to keep falling in love with my Abba more and more deeply. That is why I am on earth. Yes, I have other purposes to accomplish, serious ones, but those purposes are because he loves me and wants the best for me. He knows that when I am aligned the most closely with his purposes, the happier and more fulfilled I am, the more I feel loved and cared for by him and special to him.

A Meltdown—Off the Tracks

I suppose everyone has to find their edge and go off it. I went off mine on Tuesday, January 25th after beginning to slide the night before. In checking on the MyChart portal, I saw a message from the doctor's nurse that my scans were set on February 14, three more weeks away. That was four weeks after my first visit to UT Southwestern and almost a month and a half after receiving my diagnosis. That left me with a scary, sickening feeling. The two biggest things in dealing with cancer are timing and expertise. I felt like I traded the former for the latter. I just didn't know how to weigh all of this out. I hated the intrusion of Mark to begin with but ended up feeling certain that it was God's doing to move me in the direction of the second opinion at UT Southwestern. I also ended up feeling that my lifelong dilemma of trying to discern between God testing my surrender level and taking necessary steps to move me in a different direction to a different decision or action was a both/and this time.

I felt a crisis that I thought was easy to discern—this one was only a surrender test, and one that I failed and wept about in disappointment and fear. (Cancer brings up lots of emotions.) I decided to shut down my emotions and just resign myself to the inevitable, whatever that turned out to be. I know intellectually that I cannot see the big picture of what God is doing, but spiritual surrender was not in my deck of cards at that moment. Resignation was. I could do that one. That is how most human beings survive life anyway, especially challenging times. We just resign ourselves to the realities no matter how bleak or painful they are. I did have enough sense left to realize that I should not share my faithlessness with others for fear of hurting their faith.

I hoped to get to a better place and always do, but this time felt different. Although I wasn't angry at God exactly, I was for sure very disappointed and hurt. But no matter what, I was determined to do my best not to hurt the faith of others. That meant, like many, many other times, that I would basically be faking it. I didn't feel hypocritical about doing that. I felt like the Psalm 73 guy.

Psalm 73:13-16

[13] Surely in vain I have kept my heart pure and have washed my hands in innocence. [14] All day long I have been afflicted, and every morning brings new punishments. [15] If I had spoken out like that, I would have betrayed your children. [16] When I tried to understand all this, it troubled me deeply...

Unlike him, I did not keep my heart pure nor my hands innocent. I did feel like he did in verse 14 since receiving the news of the three week's delayed scans. But my point from the Psalm was in verses 15-16. I couldn't understand the three weeks delay, and like the Psalmist, it indeed troubled me deeply, very deeply—to the edge and off with no hope of surrender, only a grit-my-teeth-grin-and-bear-it resignation. But it was resignation to the point of trying to say what Jesus said in the Garden, "Nevertheless," and like Daniel's three friends said as they faced the fiery furnace, "Even if…" I wanted aloneness from everyone, whether they loved me or hated me. The day starting at Jewish time the prior evening and continuing to and through the next day was for me like a French movie. The French say that their movies start bad, get worse, and end! *Viva la France!*

On the evening of my very-bad-no-good-meltdown-day, I shared many of my thoughts with Theresa and was at least resigned to whatever was to come of the delayed scans and what they would eventually show. I wasn't in a good place, but I didn't think I was still in verses 21-22 of Psalm 73: "When my heart was grieved and my spirit embittered, [22] I was senseless and ignorant; I was a brute beast before you." Once again, as God often does, he exposed and embarrassed me that same evening. The protocol for tests was for a medical person to call and inform you of any scheduled scans or changes in their schedule. I had received no such calls. But for some reason, I happened to look at the portal as I was preparing to go to bed. The tests had been moved up in spite of the fact that I had been told it was impossible unless a cancellation occurred. But two tests of different types cancelled, opening up two spots on the same day at just the right intervals? How many "coincidences" could come my way in such a short span of time?

Huge Benefits of a Meltdown

After seeing the change in the schedule, I was indeed exposed and embarrassed at my lack of faith and convicted of my mistrust and accompanying sins. I stayed up for a long time, praying and journaling and reading Scripture and writing. It was a time of pain and joy uniquely mixed together in bringing my heart back to God. My lack of trust in that one twenty-four-hour period was deeply convicting and deeply saddening. Honestly, it still was when I wrote this originally. God had done nothing but bless me and show himself to me. I felt like Hagar in Genesis 16:13, "She gave this name to the LORD who spoke to her: 'You are the God who sees me,' for she said, 'I have now seen the One who sees me.'" People complain that it is difficult to believe in a God that they cannot see, much less trust him. But you can see him. He wants to be seen. He has shown himself to me over and over, but I am often too blind to see or just not paying attention. You see that in this story thus far, don't you? But in the midst of my meltdown, I didn't. And that is not nearly all that I experienced during that time, just the main points.

I continued to pursue my repentance late into the night and early the next morning. It was a rich experience. I looked up familiar passages and saw lessons I had missed before. That is a part of seeing God. He shows up in his love letter revelation, the Bible, to us in ways we haven't seen him previously. He keeps giving us new insights through both experiences and Scriptures. Romans 2:4 was one of the first verses I looked at. "Or do you show contempt for the riches of his kindness, forbearance and patience, not realizing that God's kindness is intended to lead you to repentance?" The context of this verse is showing the sins of the Jews in judging the Gentiles. They thought they had been blessed because they deserved it, that they were better than all those outside the Israelite nation. But God had been good to them to induce repentance and appreciation in them, not to exalt them. Their own judgmental attitudes condemned them.

As I thought about that context, I suddenly realized that I took it to a much higher (actually far lower) place and judged God himself! Perfectly horrific. Through his word, the sword of the Spirit (Ephesians 6:17), he cut into my messed-up heart and in the process, started his beautiful heart surgery on me. He is the Great Physician, after all. I know that God allows us to question him, just as any good parent does their children. The Psalmists prove that over and over. But the questioning can go too far, as did Job's in the Old Testament. I didn't want to cross that line, but even if I had, God would still be right there. I realized that when I began looking at the ending of Psalm 73.

Psalm 73:21-28

[21] When my heart was grieved and my spirit embittered, [22] I was senseless and ignorant; I was a brute beast before you. [23] Yet I am always with you; you hold me by my right hand. [24] You guide me with your counsel, and afterward you will take me into glory. [25] Whom have I in heaven but you? And earth has nothing I desire besides you. [26] My flesh and my heart may fail, but God is the strength of my heart and my portion forever. [27] Those who are far from you will perish; you destroy all who are unfaithful to you. [28] But as for

me, it is good to be near God. I have made the Sovereign LORD my refuge; I will tell of all your deeds.

What a beautiful ending to the Psalm! That's God in plain view. He always holds us close and holds us tight—even at our worst when we are brute beasts. God is good and always good and cannot be otherwise. In addressing the Jews in Romans 2, in spite of their sins of which they were totally unaware yet proud of and justifying, God was trying to lead them by their right hand out of the mess they were in. When we are out of our senses, God is still with us, holding us by our hands, leading us back into spiritual reality. I picture a parent with a three-year-old child who wants to go the opposite way than they are being led. They are kicking and screaming and throwing a tantrum. What does the parent do? They just keep gently pulling the child along with them in the direction they know they should go, knowing that the child will eventually give up the fight and follow, and either apologize or be taught by the parent to apologize after throwing a hissy fit. That's what good parents do and that's how children learn to trust parents. Where do parents learn how to do that? The writer of this Psalm would say, correctly, from God.

Satan's work with us is the exact same as it was with Eve in the Garden, namely, to cause us to mistrust God by believing that he is withholding something good from us; to believe that he really doesn't want the very best for us. One of his tools is to convince us that God only loves us when we are doing well. When we are a mess in a mess, he turns aside and with arms crossed in frustration or anger, he waits until we straighten up and then he turns back toward us. Then, if we have repented with enough guilt and sorrow, he is willing to give us a hug.

That is exactly the opposite of how God really works. Using the analogy of the parent holding on to their three-year-old child in rebellion, what does the parent do in this case? They hold on tighter to keep the child from hurting themselves. Now the child may step in mud puddles and skin their knees on the sidewalk in their self-inflicted escapades, but the parent holds on even tighter. Were the child not fighting, the parent could pick them up and carry them over the mud puddles and through the rough patches, but no matter what, the parent holds on – especially when the child insists on going the wrong way. That is like God, isn't it? He doesn't just hold on to us when we are gleefully following his lead. It is precisely when we are at our worst that he reaches for us. Read it.

Romans 5:6-8

⁶ You see, at just the right time, when we were still powerless, Christ died for the ungodly. ⁷ Very rarely will anyone die for a righteous person, though for a good person someone might possibly dare to die. ⁸ But God demonstrates his own love for us in this: While we were still sinners, Christ died for us.

Psalm 73 goes on to say that God keeps guiding us, teaching us and maturing us until such time as he takes us home with him to glory. Thus, as we do mature spiritually, what happens? Heaven becomes all about God and our relationship eternally with him. It's not about streets of gold or anything we humans imagine as being heaven. It's not about making 1000-yard drives on golf courses constructed from our wildest imaginations or catching ten-pound largemouth bass on every cast on the most beautiful lake imaginable. It is about being with our Abba, forever and ever, loving and being loved by him in unimaginable ways. More importantly in the here-and-now, life on earth becomes all about God and developing a relationship with him into deeper and deeper levels. Everything else in this life pales into insignificance when we get the lesson that our writer friend of Psalm 73 learned. I'm just using his words with a bit of editing. It's all right there.

He ended this marvelous chapter in this longest book in the Bible with complete satisfaction in being near God and in making him his refuge. That is all about relationship, simply and beautifully. This is why God made us and he works with us from the day of our birth until the day of our death, helping us see that and once we see it, helping us grow continually until we are at home with him. No wonder our dear writer says that he would tell the story of all of God's deeds. How could he not? He had just been led out of a dark place to the brightest realizations known to mankind. He foreshadowed the words of my favorite Bible character, the apostle Paul. "We also believe and therefore speak" (2 Corinthians 4:13).

Seeing God Everywhere

Seeing God is a learned art. It is a matter of looking and focusing. Many years ago, I was staying in the home of a good minister friend and his wife whom I had helped train. His church was conducting an evangelistic campaign, and I was the guest speaker. One afternoon, the brother and I were walking through a small grove of trees behind their house, and he commented about how the trees were just full of plums that season. I thought he was kidding me, because when I looked up into the trees I didn't see one plum. But he insisted that he wasn't joking and was surprised that I thought he was, since he assured me that the trees were indeed full of plums. I kept looking up for a while in search of plums and at a certain point, I suddenly saw them—tons of them. They were the same color as the leaves of the tree, not yet being in the ripened stage. I was shocked, pleasantly so. I just wasn't focused and prepared to see what was abundantly obvious all the time. You get the point, I'm sure. Start looking. God is everywhere, omnipresent

we say, and all loving, which means that he is in your life too—
and observably so if you are prepared to see him.

One of my "impossible" prayers for 2022 was to eliminate
negative thinking by looking at best case scenarios rather than
worst case scenarios, and to see positive ways of viewing things
that appear negative. In other words, trust that every dark cloud
has a silver lining if we will but look for it and be patient as we
look. It often takes time to see it. Hindsight is much clearer
than foresight. I think back to an unusual episode in November 2021. I had just returned from attending and speaking on
a beautiful memorial service for one of my heroes, Ron Brum-
ley, in San Diego. On the following Saturday, I was spending
time with Theresa and all was well with my world—until it
wasn't. I started having some odd little hallucinations, like I
was dropping off to sleep and having a series of quick dreams.
Yet I was wide awake and walking around inside the house and
even outside once to check the mail. I talked to Theresa about
it and we decided it was probably wise to visit the Emergency
Room, although the episode only lasted five or ten minutes.
Once there, they started doing tests of several types, primarily
checking to see if I had suffered a stroke. I hadn't. But the blood
test showed a kidney problem, serious enough to be called an
"acute kidney injury."

They checked me into the hospital for the night and hooked
me up to an IV. By morning, my kidney function was back in
the normal range. I described every part of my activities for the
past week to the doctors and nurses, including the trip to San
Diego. Dehydration was a part of the issue, I'm sure, and I had
a theory about what else might have contributed to the odd
and scary episode. None of the medical folks had any better
theories than I did, and the hospitalist discharged me just after
noon the next day.

That experience bothered me until I had my scans for

cancer explained. They injected me with Iodine-containing contrast medium in both types of scans. My specialist had my kidney function tested again before the scans, because the scan processes put a strain on the kidneys. Mine checked out fine. So, what was the silver lining in that November cloud experience? I had done something that temporarily affected my kidney function and without the strange episode, what was called an injury might have progressed to the permanent damage stage. That was a heck of a way to find it out, but a part of an ongoing roller coaster ride with an adventuresome God. At least, that is the best I can make of it, and that is good enough for me.

A Later Series of *Coincidences*

I could go on and on about that sequence of experiences and seeing God in them, but I will just include one more that I thought of when writing this initially. It's worth the read, trust me. Years ago, while living in Boston, we had a very close relationship with a couple originally from Australia, Graham and Suzanne Gumley. Graham was (and is) one of the foremost microsurgeons in the world. When they were in Boston, Graham was a professor in the medical schools of Harvard and Northeastern. They are back in Australia now, and prior to going back, Graham served as the chief surgeon in a hospital in Phnom Panh, Cambodia, a project of HOPE *Worldwide,* an organization dedicated to serving the poor and needy. With all of the injuries still occurring from Pol Pot's buried land mines, it would be interesting to hear Graham's surgical stories from that decade of his life. He has been a professor in medical schools in his home country and up to age 70, was still conducting surgeries to reattach body parts severed through accidents. I know some of those stories but won't take the time here to tell them, though they are beyond fascinating.

After years of not connecting with the Gumleys, I just

"happened" to receive an email from Graham on December 30th of 2021, the day after the sample tissue was taken by my doctor that led to the cancer diagnosis. When I communicated back via email the next day, I described in some detail my health issues, including the fact that I was awaiting the results of that test from the day prior to his first email. His reply to mine arrived January 6th, the day after I got the cancer diagnosis. In it, he asked if we could share a Zoom call to catch up, which we did a few days later, and had a wonderful talk. Graham isn't just a great surgeon; he is a great person and great disciple of Jesus. His wife is just as special.

Here's the kicker. Graham was in his office when we were talking on Zoom. He said that literally right next door to where he was sitting was the best colorectal department in all of Australia and he could ask his friends there any question that I might have or get any advice I might want. It's just one more of the incredible adventures in my spiritual roller coaster ride with God, who himself obviously loves adventures. He created us, didn't he? After hearing about one 33-day adventure in my life experience, isn't it pretty clear that God not only wants to be seen but can be seen—*clearly*? Of course, I could mention that 33 is my all-time favorite number. My email addresses both start with gordonferguson33. Coincidence? Think what you want, but I knew before I started counting the days between January 5 and February 7 what the number was going to be. I'm not always blind or not looking. As my good friend, Steve Hiddleson, would say just about now (approvingly), I'm just getting plumb "wiggly." Join me and start looking everywhere for God. He is there, anxious to be seen and to be with you.

Chapter 3

•

(E)Motion Sickness Sometimes Comes

It is inevitably true for roller coaster aficionados that thrill rides are at their best when they give you surprises. One surprise can be motion sickness to the point that you lose your breakfast, lunch or dinner upon disembarking! With God being both the designer of life's roller coaster and the one at the controls, we should expect to encounter rides replete with surprises. Sometimes those surprises are initially delightful and sometimes they are initially disappointing, occasionally devastatingly so. I was yet to experience a devastating disappointment that almost made me physically sick to my stomach; it certainly made me emotionally sick at heart. You will likely assume what the nature of my disappointment was, but you won't get that part right until you finish reading this chapter. But it was for me a devastating experience that put me back in the pits. God knows that we can never appreciate the exhilarations of life without visiting the pits occasionally at least.

An Ice Storm? Really?

After the exhilarating revelation that my very important test series was amazingly moved up from February 14 to February 3, I was relieved and elated. Peace had arrived, so I put in a period. Challenge over in one regard at least. But God then said, "Oh yeah? Watch this!" As the new date of testing approached, something else also approached—the worst weather day of the year, an ice storm. "Lord, you have got to be kidding!

How can this be happening?" It quickly became obvious that driving from my house in North Dallas to the hospital near downtown Dallas was going to be literally impossible. It was predicted to start raining the evening before my scheduled test and by midnight, the temperature would start dropping into the 20s. Good grief, Charlie Brown! I thought roller coasters had some lower heights and gentler curves somewhere. Maybe so, but obviously not yet.

Being determined to take those tests, my mind started racing in looking for solutions. I thought of finding a hotel near the hospital, near enough so that I could walk to it if necessary. In looking at a map of the area, I discovered the closest hotel about a mile away and booked it for two nights. Not only was it nearby, but it was also cheap. Great! After I booked it, I decided to look at the reviews by former guests. *Uh Oh!* It was in a bad area and most reviews mentioned drug dealers and fearful nights full of loud talking by numerous people doing drug deals. Great location for my purposes, but a scary location in a bad part of town. Oh well, you can't have everything go your way, right? It was a scary place, evidently built originally as an apartment complex with lots of separate buildings containing four one-bedroom suites apiece. When I walked into the lobby to check in, I encountered a younger man, dressed in street clothes with a glock in a holster strapped to his side, a Black man for those of you with racial presuppositions. That didn't alarm me, actually. It's the hidden pistols that concern me. I asked him if he was an officer, and as expected, he answered in the affirmative. He explained that this was a rough part of town, and he did some patrolling here regularly. Those reviews weren't wrong.

The weather report was also regrettably accurate. Ice covered the roads by morning. Fortunately, some sleet had also fallen, making driving slightly more plausible. I left the hotel early, dressed warmly, determined to leave my car and walk if I couldn't drive all the way to the hospital. Having lived in Boston for sixteen years, I wasn't a novice at driving on slick roads and I managed to make it all the way to the hospital without incident. My worst fears were of other drivers who didn't have the same experiences of driving on frozen roads that I had. But only a few brave (or not-too-bright) souls had ventured out, and I managed to dodge those few.

I would like to say that God finally put a period or at least a semicolon on my day once I arrived at the hospital. No chance of that. I won't go into the details, but nothing worked quite the way it should have. At one point, I ended up in the middle of a difference of opinion between my oncologist and the doctor in charge of my MRI regarding necessary preparations for the procedure. I will mention that the written instructions from the MRI department itself failed to include instructions for those preparations, which I pulled up on my phone and showed to the nurse. Oh, well… The nurses of the two doctors went back and forth to their respective doctors and me for some time until the MRI specialist finally asked to talk to me on the phone. It was a weird process which shouldn't have happened, but I finally decided to go with the MRI guy since I was in his house at the time, his department.

I stayed calm but registered my concern that a medical facility with their reputation should never have such an issue arise in the first place. No one disagreed with me, and they assured me that it would be addressed and corrected for the future. The delays involved resulted in a long day, just under seven hours, to take one blood test and two scans. But by then, I was pretty much expecting the unexpected. My thrill ride continued. Back to the hotel, I was thankful that the weather kept most people holed up inside rather than engaging in their usual activities in that place. The main roads were clear enough by the next afternoon to drive home on mostly clear roads, although the news stations were repeatedly urging people not to drive unless absolutely necessary. For me, it was absolutely necessary. I had had enough—time to go home, and I did.

Good News (Until it Wasn't)!

Modern technology has its positive and negative aspects. Test results, even from complicated tests, often come "stat" (immediately) and appear on the medical facility's internet portal. After my first scan on that icy day, I was reading the test results on my phone while awaiting my second scan. All of that medical jargon unsettles me, but I can usually get the main gist of what is being said. In this case, it appeared that no cancer had been detected, at least as best I could tell from a layman's perspective. Then came the cancer-detection blood test, followed by my second scan. After the tests were finished, I looked at all of the results. My best guess was that I didn't have cancer, and the next day, that guess was confirmed as true. Good news! Great news!

My first assumption was that the multitude of prayers for my healing had been answered in the affirmative. I posted the results to all of my Facebook friends and passed it on in various ways to my non-FB friends. I was ecstatic and shed many tears of joy as I poured out my gratitude to God in prayer. Here is an excerpt of my Facebook post after receiving the good news.

> None of the tests showed any cancer. The doctor is looking for answers, requesting the actual pathology slides to have her pathology department read them. She is also having me see a surgeon to examine me and make sure there is no suspicious tissue that could later develop into cancer. For them, it is understandably a mystery. Not for me. Your prayers moved God and he answered them. He

doesn't always answer with a yes and one day he will have to say no to other prayers to sustain my life, but not this time. I have been waiting to have more information before posting an update. I have it and now you have it. May God bless each of you in unexpected ways, as he has me.

The doctor's request for the slides from my previous provider was actually prompted by me in a message I sent her through the internet portal. She and my medical team had already accepted the results of the tests and had put me on a schedule of check-ups at three-month intervals. In my message, I mentioned the possibility of the cancerous tissue perhaps having been inadvertently removed by my previous surgeon in her last tissue removal for testing. That made logical sense to me, explaining both the cancer present in the tissue and not in my body. That set things in motion quickly, with "Doctor Harvard" obtaining those slides from my previous surgeon. Once the slides were reexamined, the cancer was present as expected, but no margins were found.

That being the case, I was referred to a surgeon to take a closer look and have another tissue sample tested. Once again, the cancer showed up, although it was seemingly confined to a small space and had not spread. Their concern was not only what was discovered, but what might have been present and not discovered—microscopic cancer cells in the surrounding area. Thus, the next step recommended was to have the area treated with both radiation and chemotherapy. That was the original recommendation before I went to UT Southwestern, so we hadn't lost any ground in spite of how it felt. We had probably gained ground by discovering more about the cancer, making the chemo treatment supposedly milder than the other medical oncology practice had described.

Understanding the Mystery of Miracles

Miracles have more than one definition. Most think of them as instantaneous and otherwise impossible changes, like the healings we read about in the earthly ministry of Jesus. I call these direct miracles. Then we have what I call providential miracles. These can be identified as events that could not have occurred coincidentally but had to be orchestrated by God in his providential working together of the details. The old saying that the devil is in the details is an interesting concept and can be true when humans make bad choices. But mark this down as an absolute certainty: God is in the details. I have always felt that providential miracles were the greatest type. Just doing a direct miracle instantaneously is impressive, and I do believe that God still does those at times. But for me, I am more impressed with providential miracles, for they involve humans with freedom of choice and details too intricate to even grasp.

In my initial cancer free diagnosis, I wasn't sure which category the apparent healing miracle fit. I had that one plausible explanation involving what would have been an inadvertent removal of the cancer by my first surgeon in collecting tissue for pathology. That would have fallen into the providential miracle category. And then, of course, the other possibility would have involved a direct miracle. I didn't care which it was at the time. Hearing "no cancer" was enough for me.

The Nature of My Disappointment

If you assumed that the disappointment was finding out I still had cancer after three tests saying otherwise, you would assume wrongly. Oddly, the diagnosis of cancer was not that big a deal to me. Quite a number of other diagnoses would have hit me emotionally a lot harder than a cancer diagnosis. I'm not quite sure why that is the case, but it was from the beginning. Maybe it's because I know a number of cancer survivors, although my father and many other relatives and friends have died from cancer. Maybe it's because I had lived my fourscore years already, counting my time in my mother's womb. I was old enough to die at what most would consider a "ripe old age." So grateful for that fact. Really grateful. Really blessed.

In this situation described, my biggest disappointment was informing hundreds or thousands of people who had prayed for me that the "no cancer" diagnosis had proved to be premature and inaccurate. By announcing the "no cancer" test results, many people who had prayed for me were using the term "miraculous" in answer to their prayers. Honestly, we need to believe in the power of prayer to move God to answer them, at times answering miraculously. I didn't want the reversal in diagnosis to hurt the faith of those dear to me, to put it bluntly. I prayed that this "partial" reversal didn't discourage any who had prayed and would continue to pray for me. As it turned out, their prayers would be needed far more when my roller coaster ride came to a dead halt on the precipice of eternity, which Part Two of the book describes.

I was at that point holding on to the principle mentioned earlier: building faith demands testing faith. I can handle that truth. I've had lots of practice through eight decades of life, most of those decades spent walking with God. I understand the principle and the process—most of the time, at least in looking back at it. My hindsight is better than my foresight, to be sure, but somewhere in the process, the light bulb comes back on and I see clearly once again. I greatly appreciate all of the prayers offered for my health challenge, pre-diagnosis and post-diagnosis. I believe they made a difference. The tests could have shown a much more aggressive form of cancer and one that had spread throughout my body. Although I dreaded the upcoming treatments with their potential side effects, the prognosis was good. I had faith that the cancer would be eradicated. For me, those back-and-forth diagnoses had been going on for months. I was used to them and probably need to remain used to them. I just didn't want others to be hurt or disappointed. I want to help us all to develop a bigger picture of life and death, eventually both mine and yours.

The Most Basic Principle

I mentioned earlier a principle that might have been passed over too briefly. The principle begins with the premise that life on planet earth is not only brief but highly significant—a preparation ground for eternity with God. This being true, God is constantly attempting to mold us into his own character so that heaven might be, well, heaven, with like-minded beings totally connected. This developmental process centers around building faith in a God who is good and only good, and whose love for us is unfathomable. But how does that faith come and then become a growing process through all the days of our lives? It must be tested over and over and over. The testing process is the fundamental method of developing and strengthening our faith. Hence my use of the roller coaster ride analogy. I know of none better, at least to me as a lover of roller coasters.

I keep making one fundamental mistake in how I view this most basic principle. It provides a life lesson with many applications. I keep putting periods when God is using commas. That's what we do in the midst of struggles. We see the struggle as the final result, and it ain't good! All the while God is saying, "Patience, patience—we aren't done yet; the solution is coming, and you will get through it." In my early cancer experience, I would get past one challenge, a scary part of the ride, sometimes absolutely terrifying, and want to put a period on it. End of ride. Challenge met and challenge over. I keep making that mistake. Don't you? But when we do that, we forget the principle—God builds faith precisely by testing it. And that principle demands a constant series of commas, not periods. Let's just be happy to see the occasional semicolon when the challenges are spaced out with some needed pauses inserted to allow us time to process the challenges and get ready for the next one. God knows exactly what he is doing in your life. Chill out and try to enjoy the ride. You are strapped in with him as your safety belt. You will be jerked halfway out of your seat at times, but the safety belt will never break.

Looking for the Big Picture View

No human being has all of the answers to life, nor to death. I can explain why bad things happen to good people, at least reasonably well on an intellectual basis. But when you are the one to whom bad things happen unexplainably, emotional understanding and acceptance becomes the real challenge. No pat answers will do in those moments, nor will any answers totally satisfy. Much in life remains a mystery, which is why we must live by faith and not by sight (2 Corinthians 5:7). Although we are inclined to ask, "Why me?" when tragedy strikes, the Christian would do better asking, "Why not me?" We are prepared, and thus we trust by faith these statements of Paul.

Romans 14:7-9

[7] For none of us lives for ourselves alone, and none of us dies for ourselves alone. [8] If we live, we live for the Lord; and if we die, we die for the Lord. So, whether we live or die, we belong to the Lord. [9] For this very reason, Christ died and returned to life so that he might be the Lord of both the dead and the living.

2 Corinthians 5:6-9

[6] Therefore we are always confident and know that as long as we are at home in the body we are away from the Lord. [7] For we live

by faith, not by sight. [8] We are confident, I say, and would prefer to be away from the body and at home with the Lord. [9] So we make it our goal to please him, whether we are at home in the body or away from it.

Philippians 1:20-21

[20] I eagerly expect and hope that I will in no way be ashamed, but will have sufficient courage so that now as always Christ will be exalted in my body, whether by life or by death. [21] For to me, to live is Christ and to die is gain.

I well remember watching a sad but very inspirational movie. One scene in the movie was especially helpful. The movie is "Greater," and I would urge you to see it. It is a spiritual movie based on a true story, quite inspiring. The scene to which I refer is when a mother and her oldest son are talking about the death of her youngest son, the kid brother of the older son. The son in the scene was struggling mightily with his faith in God and expressing his doubts angrily to his mother. She at one point simply said something to this effect: "Son, there are things we don't understand and will never understand on this side of eternity because we cannot see the big picture that God sees." A visual illustration added to the point being made. That has helped me more than I would have imagined, including in my cancer struggle. I don't ask "Why?" much anymore, because I know I have but little slivers of the big picture. God has it all. But prior to playing the end game and reaching home, we as believers are equipped to handle whatever challenges come our way, simply because we see enough of God to know what life is about.

The Bigger Picture...

Only God has the big picture, but we must strive to enlarge

our own picture, combining what God said in the Bible with what we allow our experiences to teach us. On January 1 of 2022, a few days before receiving my first cancer diagnosis, my home church was encouraging us to make lists of impossible prayers, miracle prayers, and I made my list. The first thing on my list was that I would not have cancer, but that if I did, it could be cured. A later item on that list involved my thinking processes, described thusly: "To eliminate negative thinking by looking at best case scenarios rather than worst case scenarios, and to see positive ways of viewing things that appear negative. If something ends up being negative, let it come as a surprise because I will be looking for best case scenarios."

After my list of impossible prayers was another list in the book we were all reading, with this subheading: "Miracle Sightings and Spiritual Insights." Near the top of that list, on Sunday, January 2, as I was anxiously (too anxiously) awaiting the initial pathology reports, I wrote this: "I may need cancer to help me spiritually or to help others through my experience. I have seen both happen with friends and heard of both happening in the lives of others many times. If this is your will, Father, please increase my faith enough to help me handle it well." This insight gave me the opportunity to put into practice the above concept of looking for best case scenarios rather than worst case ones. It took some work to get there, but by God's grace, I did (with ups and downs).

Many prayed for my healing, asking for cancer to not have the final word in what ends my life. Good prayer. I'm thankful for it. I prayed for that result too. But there are many more important aspects to the bigger picture. One may well be that I and others need spiritual healing far more than physical healing. My cancer journey took me to places with God I had never been before. My prayer is that my example will affect others similarly in their journey with him too.

I don't know all of what God has planned for this bigger picture. I know that a significant part of it involves my relationship with him. I believe that some of it includes my preparation for my eventual death, whenever and however it may come. I'll have more to say about that one in a moment. I believe that some of that bigger picture involves how my having cancer will affect others in various ways. During my early treatment scheduling, I received a call from a woman at the medical center to set up an appointment with my chemotherapy specialist. We talked for 30 minutes, not a normal conversation for her, I am sure. I started a spiritual discussion that took on a life of its own. It ended up with me going to my appointment (of which she was a part) and my giving her two of my books, one of which she had requested. During the appointment discussing the technicalities of chemo treatment, she shared what she and I had talked about with the doctor, which pulled him into the discussion. Where will that all lead? I don't know, but God knows.

Then a few days later, I went in for my final scan, a mapping scan to help determine exactly where the radiation treatments would be aimed. This visit began with a nurse collecting my vitals. Then came the IV nurse to puncture my arm once more. Then another person to explain and have me sign permission documents. (Does anyone actually read those?) Then came the two scan specialists to put me in that big apparatus, explain the process and carry it out. Then came my oncologist's PA and finally the oncologist herself. Maybe there were more procedures. Starting spiritual conversations is second nature to me, and I did it repeatedly with everyone who had to deal with me, or nearly everyone. What will come of that? I don't know, but God knows. How many people have I shared my faith with as a result of developing cancer? How many will I yet share my faith with due to experiencing cancer? Do you not think this is all a part of God's bigger picture?

In the early stages of having cancer, I wrote the remainder of this paragraph. So how bad is it to still have cancer? Gee, I don't know that it is bad at all. It has already accomplished some really good things in my life with God. I wouldn't give them up to be rid of the cancer, that much I know for sure. I also know that many spiritual seeds are being sown with many different medical people. One of them may wake up one morning facing the biggest challenge of their life and think of the old crazy preacher guy that they just cared for recently and try to figure out how to get back in touch with me. With many of my books listed on Amazon and having two web sites, it wouldn't take a lot of effort on their parts to find me. Plus, I give out cards with my web sites and phone number listed. God does work in mysterious ways, his wonders to perform. I love that old hymn with those words in it, and I love having seen God do it in my life, time and time again. There is a much bigger picture than we now see, but I have no doubt that God will keep revealing more of it to us, especially if we are looking for it. There is a God who sees, wants to be seen and most certainly can be seen.

PART TWO
Sitting on the Brink of Eternity

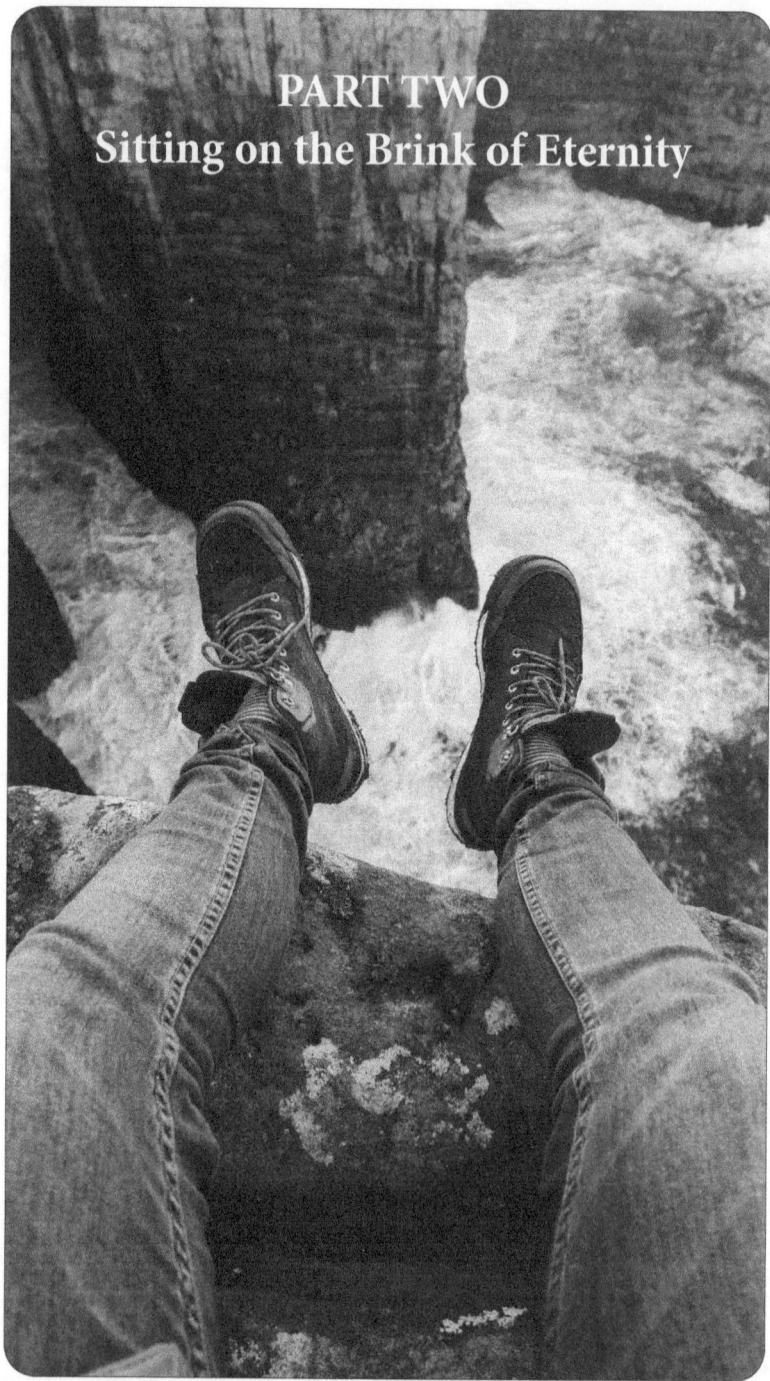

Introduction to Part Two

You might find it hard to believe, but Part One about the roller coaster ride was the tame part of my whole journey. What happened next, to continue the roller coaster analogy one last time, was like coming to what you thought was the end of the ride, only to find yourself going through one big loop after another with the g-forces leaving you feeling like you were being crushed. The upcoming chapters describe what happened and the insights I gained from the whole experience of sitting with God on the brink of eternity.

This part of the book you will find different in approach from Part One, for it was describing a three-and-a-half-month roller coaster ride from diagnosis to disaster, mostly in chronological order. Part Two describes a series of insights I received during the disaster period when in the hospital for 23 days, thinking I might well die. I don't know if any overall central theme can be found, although a number of chapters are quite related to certain other chapters covering similar themes. When facing the real possibility of death, I thought mostly about God, God and me, my family and the people with whom I came into contact who impacted my thinking. What comes to a dying man's mind? In reading Part Two, you will find out what came into my mind. Much of it just popped into my head with no connection to any current context. Surreal would be a mild word to describe it all.

It turned out that I had an enzyme deficiency that not only is very rare, but you never know you have it unless you are treated with a certain kind of chemotherapy drug. That particular drug is fairly far down the list of those most commonly used. The chances of having both the condition and being treated with that drug are one in many millions. But I was one of those few, and one who survived. Many don't. Oddly perhaps, after I understood the odds of that combination, my faith increased. God surely had to be in the middle of it. After a wild and woolly 23 day stay in the hospital, I came home and walked in with the aid of a walker. I was extremely weak throughout the whole hospital experience, unable to lift my heels from the bed. Although I had been an avid walker for years, taking three to five mile fast-paced walks at least five days per week, upon arrival at home I could barely walk across the room. My previous conditioning had disappeared completely.

One thing I could do was write, and that I did. I felt compelled to record the account of my illness and narrow escape from it, but more importantly, to describe the insights I gained during what felt to me like sitting on the brink of eternity with God. Something happened to me emotionally and spiritually that I can't really explain, but the spiritual insights I gained into myself, and God, I can explain. I presented this material initially in the form of a series of twenty video podcasts, with each episode consisting of me making a presentation in the style of a fireside chat, followed by a segment with a fellow church member asking me questions and interacting with me. The video series can be seen on YouTube under the heading of "Eternity's Brink."[ii] I and others felt the material was worth preserving in written form, hence the writing of this book. Each remaining chapter is brief, but I believe the varied topics prompted from my near-death experience are worth sharing. I would say to enjoy the ride, but now that we are on the "brink," I will just say enjoy the view!

Chapter 4

•

What in the World Just Happened?

When I received my official diagnosis of cancer on January 5, 2022, I was surprisingly not disturbed emotionally. For one thing, a preliminary diagnosis had been suggested earlier, but remained a bit uncertain for several months. Thus, it wasn't a new topic nor a surprising one. For another thing, I recalled hearing a lecture many decades ago about how stress affects the body, and I accepted the speaker's conclusions as valid. He said that stress seeks out the weakest place in the body and manifests itself there. Since I was 18 years old (during a period of high stress), I had experienced issues with the part of the body where cancer eventually did manifest itself. Thus, I pretty much expected to eventually develop cancer there. In fact, I told my surgeon and oncologist that the surprise wasn't finding out I had cancer; the surprise was that it had taken so long to develop, especially given that I am a type A (triple A actually) personality—a high stress guy. Having lived a very adventure-filled life, some of the stresses were good ones, but many were anxiety based.

After a series of interesting events about which I have written in Part One of the book, I began treatment for cancer on March 28 of 2022. For three weeks, five days a week, I had a radiation treatment and took six large chemo pills daily. In spite of all of the warnings about side effects, I had none (almost). The one exception occurred during a three mile walk near the end of the three-week period, when the ball of my right foot started hurting badly. I was at the halfway point and had to limp home very slowly, then discovering a very large blister. One of the listed potential side effects of the chemo was developing sensitivity and redness on the bottom of the feet and on the palms of the hands. But other than that, I had no side effects for those initial three weeks and congratulated myself on breezing through the treatments. Pride goes before a fall.

The Sunday following those three weeks was Easter Sunday. After enjoying a meal with our son and his family, disaster struck. I began losing my body fluids from every place where they could escape, especially at the bottom end—in violent fashion. Suffice it to say it was bad and unlike any sickness I have ever experienced in my entire life. I'm one of those people who just doesn't get sick, except very rarely. My immune system is amazingly strong. I've traveled all over the world during different kinds of flu and virus outbreaks and never caught any of it, nor have I ever taken flu shots (until 2022). But from the evening of Easter Sunday until the next morning, my well-conditioned body was drained of body fluids and strength almost completely. On that Monday morning after my "adventure" began the previous day, I had to be helped out of the car into a wheelchair to take my last radiation treatment for some weeks.

The next five days were a blur. I slept most of the time. I was severely dehydrated, and an IV administered at a medical facility on Tuesday had no positive effect on how I felt. The diarrhea was relentless. On Friday, I was back at the same medical facility and was asked a question by a Nurse Practitioner which brought me to my senses. She asked me if I thought I would be okay if I went home. She and the chemo doctor did not. It suddenly hit me that if I did go home, I would likely die. So, my wife and son and I went to the Emergency Room and I checked into the hospital for what was to become a 23 day stay.

I don't quite know how to describe what happened during

that time, although I can better describe my emotional and spiritual state after the hospital ordeal was over than I can what prompted it. I ended up in something like a state of near euphoria during the last part of my stay. Sometime in that period, I talked on the phone to my dear old friend, Tom Jones. A few weeks later he asked if I had ever considered that I might be bipolar, based on what seemed to him like a manic state on my part. I laughed and reminded him that my tendency was typically to be depressive, not manic. The euphoric state was temporary, but it was quite interesting while it lasted. I will describe later what were likely contributing factors to it.

For the first ten of those days in the hospital, I tried eating once and promptly threw it back up—with gusto! I was diagnosed with an ileus, which means my insides were locked up and not functioning normally. The doctors were reluctant to insert a PICC (peripherally inserted central catheter) and start giving me nourishment via that kind of IV (TPN—total parenteral nutrition). I had a low-grade fever, and they were concerned about an undetected infection. So, we waited and tested and waited and tested—for ten days. For most of that time, I was pretty much out of it. I was receiving fluids for hydration through an IV but remember being fixated on the idea of drinking a big Coke and a big strawberry drink from a big glass filled with ice.

I was obviously extremely thirsty. I remember thinking that if I could stay focused on quenching my thirst with those drinks that it might provide enough motivation to stay alive. Seriously. Also obviously, the thoughts of death were constantly present. I was later told that I had said at one time that I would have to get better to die. It was a very rough ten days. Joy (our daughter, the wife of our son, Bryan) took pictures of me at three different stages, and the latter two I eventually posted on Facebook. The first one was taken during that ten-day period and in it, I looked like I was dead. I didn't post that one. The first time my son came into my room and saw me in that state, he thought I must have just died. So that's what happened that led me to sitting with God on the brink of eternity.

After I survived and it was all over, I had hazy memories of procedure after procedure having been performed—X-Rays, CT scans, MRI's, shots, insertions of objects, etc. When I finally felt better, I logged into the portal and found the list of all procedures performed. I copied and pasted them into a Word document and hit the "sum" button—300 even! This doesn't include the 28 radiation treatments I received before and after my hospital stay. Just as I expected to develop cancer from my high stress level experiences and personality, I now expect to develop it again due to the high treatment level experiences. A body can take only so much, and I am amazed that I am as healthy now as I was before this journey started. But using the 80-year mark mentioned in Psalm 90, at age 81, I am now playing on company money! (Really always have been.) Thank you, Jesus!

Chapter 5

•

Face to Face with God

The nights were the worst. I was having hallucinations and delusions. I imagined myself in different places, with other people present and some really strange smells as a part of it. I couldn't sleep much at all and was thinking about death and meeting God much of the time. While I was in that condition, it brought my view of God into sharp focus. Most of my life, I have struggled with my view of God. The way I have seen him produced a fear of aging and death in me that has been very difficult to shed. I have for years explored in various ways how our view of God is developed in the first place. In the spiritual realm, little is more important than our view of God, what we believe is his view of us, and how we think the two of us should relate.

My early opinion, and a popular one, is that our view of God grows out of our view of our fathers, if we have one at home, and if not, from our view of other male authority figures in our lives. There is unquestionably validity to this theory. I remember counseling a brother who grew up with a very domineering, harsh father. His view of God was obviously faulty, based on clear evidence in his life. I once asked him to take a week and come back with a very specific description of how he viewed God. He basically described God as what we call the "Clockmaker God." In other words, God did create the world (wound it up to start it ticking) but has nothing to do with us besides watch what we do. He is uninvolved in our lives physically and emotionally. He watches us and will one day judge us on the basis of what he has observed in us. After this "god" was described, I asked him who it sounded like, and without hesitation, he said, "my dad."

This idea of how we develop our view of God obviously has merit and for years, I thought my view of God came in this manner. My dad was very harsh in my young, most formative years. Thankfully, when I got married at age 22, it was like Daddy took off his parent's hat and put on his friend's hat. In the decades following until his death, we were very good friends. Evidently, a part of the Ferguson family culture was that a father was responsible for his children until they were adults but not afterwards. This view would understandably have relieved a lot of Dad's stress of feeling responsible for me prior to my marriage. But what happens to children in their most formative early years does continue to affect us. Logically, my father could have been the one who strongly influenced me to see God as harsh.

However, ongoing talks with my younger sister helped me to figure out that this wasn't the case—a surprise to me. Pam and I are 10½ years different in age but think a lot the same. We definitely have a shared view of our immediate family and extended family as well. She is much nicer and gentler than I am, but we are in most ways on the same wavelength in our views. My frequent talks with her have been so helpful to me in many ways. She is a very wise and spiritual woman, the wife of a preacher. We laugh at how we grew up in a dysfunctional family, including our extended family, yet I ended up a preacher and she ended up married to one. God has his ways, often mysterious ways, as the old hymn words it.

Through our talks, I eventually figured out where my view of God originated, and it wasn't our dad. There are two parts to this discovery. The first came to me when I pictured myself as a small child in the little church we attended. My dad came to church with Mother and me most of the time, but it was obvious to me even as a very young child that he was not into it. He attended to please my mother. Thus, I didn't connect him to my concept of God. I remember (still) a man in that church who was a bit rotund and very kind, and when thinking of God, I pictured his face. Although that memory was embedded in my mind rather clearly, it was also embedded deeply enough to take some time and real concentration to dig it out. But if my earliest view of God grew out of my view of that particular kind man, how did I end up with a harsh view of God? That's a really good question and it took me even more time to sort out the answer to that one.

The little church of which we were a part was an odd one, and legalistic to the core. My grandmother and mother bore strong witness to the truth of this statement. My grandmother dwindled down to near nothing physically before dying just short of her 89th birthday. I believe she clung to life out of fear of meeting God, given her view of him. My mother reflected the same fears. Her view of death was never like the hymn, *Safe in the Arms of Jesus*. It much more resembled the view suggested by another hymn, *There's An All-Seeing Eye Watching You*. Yes, that is a real song. Look it up on YouTube. The lyrics leave no doubt that this all-seeing eye (God) is watching you to see if you step out of line, not watching over you to protect you or love you. That was my mother's view of God, and it pervaded her religious views across the board. Plus, it transferred to me, regrettably. While I will forever be indebted to my mother for instilling in me the utmost respect for God and an unshakable trust in the Bible as the inspired word of God, my faulty view of God himself has been a burden not easily unloaded.

To give you a practical example of what this kind of viewpoint produces, let me tell you about a conversation my mother had with me about sexual morality when I was in the 8th grade. I remember the year because of how I applied the content. In our church, sexual immorality, including sex before marriage, was pretty much viewed as the "unpardonable sin." On that occasion, Mother basically explained it in much that way. If you had sex before marriage, you were destined for hell —no if's and no but's. I at once thought of my friend Ronnie. He had recently told me about having sex for the first time, and I do recall that we were in the 8th grade. I remember thinking to myself as mother continued her lecture, "Well, that's it for Ronnie. No matter what else happens the rest of his life, he is doomed to hell." As you can surmise, the doctrines of forgiveness and grace received little emphasis in our church.

Then to add to my problem while still fairly young, I attended what was called a "Preacher's School" when in my upper 20s to prepare for ministry. I loved what I learned in that school in so many ways, but we too were bent in a fairly legalistic direction. The curriculum was impressive, especially in its focus on the biblical text. We studied through the entire Bible in a verse-by-verse fashion. I learned a ton of Bible in the process and loved every minute of it. However, since we dug into the entire text of the Old Testament, given my predisposition to see God as harsh, certain accounts in the Old Testament added evidence that my view must be correct. We also studied the texts emphasizing grace, but my background blocked me from fully appreciating these types of passages. The harsh stuff stood out, and there's plenty of it in there to stand out.

I developed a sermon early on describing the different ways men sin against God, using material from the Old Testament. Here are some of the Old Testament figures mentioned in my lesson: Cain, Nadab and Abihu, King Saul, Uzzah and others. Perhaps you are familiar with the account of Korah, Dathan and Abiram where their sin led to God opening up the ground to swallow them and their entire families. No doubt the Old Testament has some scary stuff in it, and whatever one's view of God is, these accounts have to be considered and explained in a way that harmonizes with our view of the nature of God. Honestly, that is no easy task for anyone, and it has proved quite formidable for me.

Chapter 6

•

A *Personal* Relationship with God?

Religious folks often speak of having a personal relationship with God. What does that actually mean? How personal can it be? When you read those aforementioned passages from the Old Testament, it is not easy to grasp that God even wants a relationship with us that could be described as personal. To me, a personal relationship involves "warm and fuzzy" as a part of it, a feeling of closeness in which hugs (and maybe kisses) would be expected and enjoyed. Can we have that with God? Does he even want that? I know he wants us to fear and reverence him, for the Old Testament makes that abundantly clear, but what about the personal part? Maybe those questions don't come into your mind. If not, good for you. They do come into my mind, which you can surely understand by knowing my background with its challenges.

Answers have come to me in stages in a variety of different ways. One of the early stages was when I developed my teaching materials on the Book of Romans. This stage started early, for I originally developed a course on Romans in my early 30's when teaching in the same Preacher's School I had graduated from a few years prior. I became "the" Romans teacher in the school and taught the course repeatedly. It was pretty much the same material later found in my early booklet, "Justified," and still later expanded into my book, *Romans: The Heart Set Free*.[iii]

Interestingly, the title of the booklet encapsulates almost the whole story of grace in Christ. *Justified* translates a Greek legal term that means "not guilty" or "innocent." I describe justified as meaning "just-as-if-I'd never sinned." Through the years as I taught Romans many times in many places, my view of God was pretty much on target. Some of the illustrations I "stole" from others and included in my printed offerings thrill my heart and bring tears to my eyes every time I read them. Through the eyes of Romans, grace abounds and is everywhere to be found!

In my later years, I've not taught Romans much, which has been a recent realization. As a partial result, I have struggled more with my view of God and moved back toward my early tendencies. But God allows struggles for a reason. I believe he wanted me to look for and find other ways to deepen my faith in him, his grace and his personal interest in me as his son. Maybe that's why I ended up in the hospital. One example may leave you scratching your head—or not. I woke up one day a few years back just feeling the need for a hug from God. He is said to be our Abba, our Dad, and I needed a Daddy hug. We were at our little cottage near a lake in East Texas, where we spent a lot of time after we bought it in the summer of 2016. It was a great place for writing, and I wrote several books and many articles while looking out the windows at the lake across the street. The pandemic increased our time at the lake.

Anyway, that particular morning when I felt a strong need for a hug from God, I started thinking about ways he would give hugs. The most obvious is when he hugs us through other people. I often tell people that whatever love they feel from me, multiply it a million times and they will begin to grasp how much God loves them. He uses people as vessels to express his love, but it must be multiplied many, many times to get the real picture. When God uses others to talk to me, write to me, or literally to hug me, I often am attuned spiritually enough to the spirit world to realize that it is God giving me a hug. But how else does God give hugs? Answering prayers with a yes would be another way but there are yet others.

The way I am going to describe in the following example I would have questioned earlier in life and probably have thought it just weird. That morning, as I said, I really wanted to see or feel God. I happened to look down on the floor of our bedroom at an air vent that delivered warm air in the winter and cool air in the summer. It was summertime and the air from that vent was blowing right in my face when I was sleeping. I was good with the warm air in my face during the winter, but the cold air bothered me. I started thinking about how to solve that problem.

I could just put a cardboard box in front of it to block the airflow, but I thought some customized solution likely existed if I could just think of it. I decided to go out into the garage and see if any answer made itself evident. As I opened the back door of the detached garage, the first thing I saw was a set of shelves where I stored all sorts of things. The first shelf my eye focused on held a plastic container that I didn't remember seeing before. I immediately thought about the air vent and its size. I grabbed the plastic container and went quickly back inside to the bedroom. The container fit over the vent perfectly. All I had to do was cut off one end and I had a customized solution to redirect the airflow.

I didn't remember having such a container in the garage. All I know is that it was sitting in the exact place that my eyes first settled on after opening the garage door, and it was the perfect solution for my need. As soon as I saw it, I felt like I had received a hug from God. I think he somehow arranged that sequence on that day when I asked him for a hug. Does that sound crazy to you? At one time it would have to me, most definitely. But since then, I have experienced many similar instances which I believe God arranged as hugs.

Earlier in the book, I made the statement that God is a God who wants to be seen and can be seen. I used my favorite illustration about going from not seeing something to seeing it everywhere in amazing fashion—the plums example. On my teaching website (gordonferguson.org) is an article entitled, "I Have Lost My Faith (in Coincidences)."[iv] It's a long article and mentions many of the events in my life prior to becoming a preacher. It actually forms an unusual prequel to my book, *My Three Lives*,[v] and is interesting for that reason alone. But the overall emphasis of the article is that I believe God is with me and in my life every day, all day, and has been my entire life, even during the years when I wasn't close to seeking him or anything godly. Some days I "see" him; most days I do not. But he is there whether I see him or not. I love the days when I see him and feel him, and I'm quite sure he shares the same sentiment with me.

Relationship is definitely the operative word. I remember an occasion when I was thinking about the various terms in the Bible which describe God. Many terms are used to describe him, many of which focus only on his power and authority. These don't bring a relationship to mind, at least not a warm, close personal relationship. Then what should have been obvious hit me. Prior to conversion, we have a Creator/created relationship with God. He wants it to be much more than that, and in fact he provided great motivation to bring it about by becoming a man to die for those whom he created. That's the gospel story, which is too beautiful to be believed, yet it is true, and God somehow enables us to believe it. Other religions have the concept of their gods visiting planet earth in human form, as Acts 14 illustrates, but Christianity is absolutely unique in the concept of the Creator dying for the created. Simply astounding!

Friends With God—Really?

How can we view God as a Friend when he is also the Judge of all mankind? How can we view him as Abba Father, when he is the Almighty God of creation, omniscient (all-knowing), omnipotent (all-powerful), omnipresent (ever-present everywhere), and omnibenevolent (perfect in his goodness and love)? Good questions, right? God demands and deserves the utmost respect and reverence, and many passages could be quoted to demonstrate this truth. However, once we are converted and become spiritual re-creations of God, the relationship becomes far, far different.

Perhaps a human illustration can help us. While there is nothing about me (a sinner) that deserves significant levels of respect, leadership roles in which I have functioned do. When I am functioning in those roles, some typically don't know me in a personal way, and some know me at a deep level as close friends. Functioning in a role that carries authority should cause everyone in that setting to show proper respect to me as I am active in that role. I cannot be teaching the Bible and have a close friend interrupting me or otherwise deterring me from the task at hand, and a real friend would never do that. (1 Corinthians 14:34-35, properly understood contextually, makes this point well as Paul instructed wives to stop interrupting their prophesying husbands by asking questions. They were told to wait and ask them at home.)

But when my teaching session ends, let's picture two of those in the class coming over to my house afterwards, one a close friend and the other someone who doesn't know me outside the teacher/student relationship. As they come inside my house, each of the two would view me and relate to me differently at the outset. One would be very relaxed and conversing with me as good friends do, while the other one would probably be a bit uncertain about how to relate to me in the beginning. They would be paying close attention to me in trying to determine what my expectations of them were. Is it going to remain a teacher/student relationship or become something else? If I am like Jesus, I will do my best to put them at ease as quickly as possible and establish a friend-to-friend relationship with them.

I remember going golfing with a much younger minister (Steve Hiddleson, whom I mention elsewhere in the book) who was new to the staff and had no personal relationship with me prior to that outing. He nervously explained that he had listened to many of my audio lessons and felt intimidated to be in this casual setting with me as we teed off on the first hole. I just laughed and said, "As poorly as I play, you will lose that feeling by the third hole!" That put him at ease and by the end of the round, we had already made good progress toward building a personal friendship and went on to become great friends despite our age and role differences. That is exactly what I wanted to see happen.

I don't want anyone to ever feel intimidated by my age or role or anything else. I make every effort to dispel such feelings in those who are just starting to get acquainted with me and am pretty good at doing so. When I am functioning in a role that necessitates being somewhat of an authority figure, I want to leave that behind when I step down from my teaching platform. At that point, I am just one of the bros. Bottom line, I want to be friends with people and never have them put me on any type of pedestal.

I believe God wants us to show him the utmost respect and reverence because that is what we, his creatures, need. Proverbs 1:7 is clear regarding this need: "The fear of the LORD is the beginning of knowledge, but fools despise wisdom and instruction." But I also believe that God wants us to relax and be his friend. The settings we are in and the people we are with will affect how we respond in his presence, but underneath it all, friendship remains. We are never disrespectful or irreverent in his presence, but we should never be governed by fear of the wrong type. "There is no fear in love. But perfect love drives out fear, because fear has to do with punishment. The one who fears is not made perfect in love" (1 John 4:18).

I love this statement of Jesus in John 15:15: "I no longer call you servants, because a servant does not know his master's business. Instead, I have called you friends, for everything that I learned from my Father I have made known to you." The two greatest leaders in the formation of Israel were said to be friends of God. Abraham was called God's friend because of his faith (James 2:23). "The LORD would speak to Moses face to face, as one speaks to a friend" (Exodus 33:11). Let's join them in being friends with God! As we work to carry out what we call the Great Commission (Co-mission, us and him), Jesus finishes up Matthew 28 with this very appropriate promise: "And surely I am with you always, to the very end of the age."

What does friendship mean to you? Although there are many types and levels of friendship, the most important one is well described in Proverbs 18:24 as the friend who sticks closer than a brother. Whoever else fits into that definition for you, I know God does. The old hymn, *My God and I,* is on target in describing the possibilities in having a real friendship with God. Just listen to these words and picture them taking place with you and God.

> My God and I go in the fields together,
> We walk and talk as good friends should and do;
> We clasp our hands, our voices ring with laughter,
> My God and I walk through the meadow's hue.
>
> He tells me of the years that went before me,

When heavenly plans were made for me to be;
When all was but a dream of dim conception,
To come to life, earth's verdant glory see.

My God and I will go for aye together,
We'll walk and talk as good friends should and do;
This earth will pass, and with it common trifles,
But God and I will go unendingly.

During those long nights in the hospital, God and I were friends. I saw him as a friend, and I talked with him as a friend. That's why I chose the initial title for the podcast series, "Sitting with God on the Brink of Eternity." That's exactly what it felt like. I didn't know whether I was about to enter it with him or not, but we talked about it. Sometimes I wanted to go and sometimes I wanted to stay, but even when I wanted to stay (for the sake of my wife and family), I realized that if I did, I would likely have to go through another time like that one to escape this planet. We all die. God and I ended our conversations much the same every night. I said that he knew what I couldn't know, as Psalm 139:16 states: "all the days ordained for me were written in your book before one of them came to be." Therefore, since knowing the time and circumstances of my death is beyond my pay grade, I just told him that I would try to get some sleep and let him worry about it (not that he worries). I think those times provided pretty good examples of real friendship.

Chapter 7

•

Finding Clarity in See God

Most importantly, the Bible itself shows the type of relationship that God longs for with us. Many passages could be quoted to prove that point. Here are just a few of them, many taken from the Old Testament, for reasons you can probably guess.

[17] "The LORD your God is with you, the Mighty Warrior who saves. He will take great delight in you; in his love he will no longer rebuke you, but will rejoice over you with singing." (Zephaniah 3:17)

[15] "But you, Lord, are a compassionate and gracious God, slow to anger, abounding in love and faithfulness." (Psalm 86:15)

[15] "Can a mother forget the baby at her breast and have no compassion on the child she has borne? Though she may forget, I will not forget you! [16] See, I have engraved you on the palms of my hands; your walls are ever before me." (Isaiah 49:15-16)

[7] "How priceless is your unfailing love, O God! People take refuge in the shadow of your wings. [8] They feast on the abundance of your house; you give them drink from your river of delights. [9] For with you is the fountain of life; in your light we see light." (Psalm 36:7-9)

[22] "Because of the LORD's great love we are not consumed, for his compassions never fail. They are new every morning; great is your faithfulness." (Lamentations 3:22-23)

³ "The LORD appeared to us in the past, saying: "I have loved you with an everlasting love; I have drawn you with unfailing kindness." (Jeremiah 31:3)

³⁷ "No, in all these things we are more than conquerors through him who loved us. ³⁸ For I am convinced that neither death nor life, neither angels nor demons, neither the present nor the future, nor any powers, ³⁹ neither height nor depth, nor anything else in all creation, will be able to separate us from the love of God that is in Christ Jesus our Lord." (Romans 8:37-39)

¹ "See what great love the Father has lavished on us, that we should be called children of God! And that is what we are! (1 John 3:1)

⁸ "...God is love." (1 John 4:8)

¹⁹ "We love because he first loved us." (1 John 4:19)

⁴ "But because of his great love for us, God, who is rich in mercy, ⁵ made us alive with Christ even when we were dead in transgressions—it is by grace you have been saved. ⁶ And God raised us up with Christ and seated us with him in the heavenly realms in Christ Jesus, ⁷ in order that in the coming ages he might show the incomparable riches of his grace, expressed in his kindness to us in Christ Jesus." (Ephesians 2:4-7)

¹⁶ "I pray that out of his glorious riches he may strengthen you with power through his Spirit in your inner being, ¹⁷ so that Christ may dwell in your hearts through faith. And I pray that you, being rooted and established in love, ¹⁸ may have power, together with all the Lord's holy people, to grasp how wide and long and high and deep is the love of Christ, ¹⁹ and to know this love that surpasses knowledge—that you may be filled to the measure of all the fullness of God" (Ephesians 3:16-19)

One of my favorite demonstrations of God's love for us is found in Luke 15 in the account of the Prodigal Son. To really get the point, you must understand that the father in the story represents God, and then you need to put yourself back into that cultural setting. When the younger son asked for his inheritance while his father was yet alive, that was not just disrespectful; it brought shame upon the father. Then the shame was compounded when the son started using his inheritance to live in open sin and rebellion, in Gentile territory at that. The older brother's comments in the story show that bad news travels fast and everyone, including the father's friends, surely knew of the disgraceful behavior of the younger son. But finally, the boy had enough of living in the pig pen and decided to come home. His expectations were in line with how the average father of that day would have responded to the same situation. If he allowed a rebellious son to come back at all, it would have been as a servant, an act designed to bring disgrace to the one who had disgraced him. There would have been nothing shown in their interactions suggesting a father/son relationship, at least not initially and probably not ever.

The returning son in the story understood the culture and what should happen in his case. But the father in the story was not of this earth; he was the heavenly Father. What did he do? Previously, as much as he loved the son, he did not go and try to talk him out of the pig pen. God will not violate the freedom of choice that he has given us, even when we use it badly. But this father was looking down the road constantly, hoping against hope that the boy would come to his senses and return home. When he spotted the boy walking hesitantly and ashamedly toward the house, the father was filled with compassion, not with the anger that a mere human father would have felt after being repeatedly shamed by his offspring. This Father then ran to greet him rather than waiting for the kid to come to him and humble himself before him as would have been expected. Someone wrote a book about this Bible account and entitled it, "Will God Run?" Obviously, the answer is yes—a thousand times, yes! His pursuit of us is relentless.

The boy had his repentance story well-rehearsed. It had three parts. He only got the first two parts out before being interrupted by the God of all grace. "But the father said to his servants, 'Quick! Bring the best robe and put it on him. Put a ring on his finger and sandals on his feet.'" From there, the celebration party was set in motion, and given who was throwing the party, it would have been quite a party. But what we must not miss is that even before the runaway started confessing his repentance, before he got one word out, his father hugged and kissed him. What does this tell you about the kind of relationship God wants with you and me? A ton. He wants it to be a warm and fuzzy relationship, and any view of God that does not include this fact cannot be correct. But there is more—much, much more. The next chapter reveals what was for me the most significant insight I had during my whole ordeal about the nature of God.

Chapter 8

•

A Beautiful Realization

How do you know a person, really know them? This knowledge can come through several avenues. One is through their actions. "By their fruit you will recognize them. Do people pick grapes from thornbushes, or figs from thistles? [17] Likewise, every good tree bears good fruit, but a bad tree bears bad fruit. [18] A good tree cannot bear bad fruit, and a bad tree cannot bear good fruit" (Matthew 7:16-18). Our actions begin to define us early in life, as Proverbs 20:11 informs us. "Even small children are known by their actions, so is their conduct really pure and upright?" The challenge of defining God by his actions we have already mentioned. Some of those actions seem scarily harsh and some seem tender and warm. Therefore, trying to really grasp the nature of God through examining his actions alone falls short of the goal, at least for me.

The same challenge exists when looking at the titles or names of God. This could be a long study if we considered all of the Hebrew terms thus used, so let's just look at some we have already mentioned. Creator, Lord, King, Judge, Father, Abba, Friend. These also provide us with a bit of a mixed bag. Understanding that the three latter terms are covenant terms for those in a saved relationship with God is helpful, but terminology and titles alone don't fully clarify the nature of God for me. More is needed. What is the essence of God's nature? What best defines him? Who is our God, *really*?

Now we come to what I believe to be the main revelation God brought to my mind during my hospital struggles. It may well have been the reason he allowed me to go through those struggles in the first place. If so, it was worth it. I believe the implications and applications of this one point about the nature of God are absolutely monumental. Yet, it is clearly stated in the Bible although most people simply miss the point, amazingly. It is an obvious truth hidden in plain sight! For me, it began with one little statement coming to mind made years ago by an old friend named Jim McGuiggan. Jim is one of the most interesting, captivating people I have ever had discussions with, and we had a number of them. We both were teachers at Preacher's Schools, two of the best-known ones, and this shared profession brought us together on occasion.

I have long felt that Jim was perhaps the most outstanding Bible scholar in the mainstream Churches of Christ in earlier days. His study was broad and his presentations of it were captivating, whether in print or in speech (with his Irish brogue). He wrote both New Testament and Old Testament commentaries, with some of the latter exegeting several of the most challenging Old Testament prophetical books. His commentary on Ezekiel[vi] is my go-to source when trying to figure out the meanings of what I believe to be the most difficult book to interpret in the Old Testament (actually, in the entire Bible). He wrote extensively on prophecy and exposed the errors of modern "end-times" teachers. His book, *The Reign of God*[vii] is priceless in expanding one's view of God. But in spite of his extensive writing about complex doctrinal topics, his books containing short devotional chapters about our relationship to God and each other are my favorites. The titles of two in this genre give insight into the contents: *The God of the Towel*[viii] and *Jesus, Hero of Thy Soul.*[ix]

Before we proceed with my recall of his little statement, let me ask you a question. Suppose you were a part of a very large church which had many ministers on the staff of the church. What if someone asked you which one of the ministers was the very best one and to describe them with one word or a very brief phrase. What might you say makes them the best in your opinion? Some common answers could be along these lines. He's a great speaker. He's a really effective organizer. He's always nice to me and others I see him interact with. He has a good marriage and family. He knows his Bible extremely well. He connects with the audience and with individuals on an emotional level. He has both intellectual and emotional intelligence. Just what might you say about your favorite minister right now in describing why they are your favorite? I know how God would both identify and describe the best one on any church staff anywhere. I do. Unquestionably. Jesus said it.

This leads us to the statement that came to mind as I was somewhere between life and death in that hospital bed. Here it is: "God did not become a servant when he became a man; he became a man precisely because he was a servant." I immediately thought of Matthew 20:25-28. "Jesus called them together and said, 'You know that the rulers of the Gentiles lord it over them, and their high officials exercise authority over them. 26 Not so with you. Instead, whoever wants to become great among you must be your servant, 27 and whoever wants to be first must be your slave—28 just as the Son of Man did not come to be served, but to serve, and to give his life as a ransom for many.'" Jesus uses two terms to differentiate between spiritual leadership and worldly leadership. All spiritual leaders are to be servants (*diakonos*), and the greatest of them are to be slaves (*doulos*). Assuming the position of a slave meant to renounce all individual rights, and to live one's life in the service of others.

In Matthew 23, Jesus was condemning the leadership of the Pharisees and teachers of the law in no uncertain terms. He forbad applying titles to mere men, leaders or not. As I explain in the first chapter of my book, *Dynamic Leadership*,[x] we can be rightly described in terms of function and role, but never in terms of titles and offices. I am not Gordon the Teacher (with a capital "T"), but Gordon who teaches, and unless I am functioning in that role, I am just one of the brothers—on level ground at the foot of the cross with everyone else. Just before Jesus pronounced his seven woes upon the leaders of his day, he said about the same thing he had said to the apostles with their worldly views of leadership. [11] "The greatest among you will be your servant. [12] For those who exalt themselves will be humbled, and those who humble themselves will be exalted" (Matthew 23:11-12).

I have probably written more about spiritual leadership than any other biblical subject, and yet I think very few church leaders understand what Jesus is teaching in these two accounts in Matthew. We cannot seem to expunge our worldly views of leadership. We simply cannot, at least the large majority cannot. If you are shocked by my dogmatism here, let me illustrate. A dear sister of mine, a former ministry staff member herself, shared an experience she had that didn't shock me, but it saddened me. She listened to recordings of the majority of the main lessons delivered at one of our conferences—one held in 2016 in St. Louis. She was especially struck with how the various speakers introduced themselves.

All but one did it something like this: "Hello, my name is _____, and my wife and I lead the _____ church." The one exception evidently took Matthew 20 literally and said: "Hello, my name is Tom Brown, and my wife and I *serve* the North River church." I'm not surprised that Tom was the one who took this approach. It was his spirituality and humility that drew me and my wife into this family of churches back in the early 1980's. In the classes of the recent church Summit

Conference in Orlando, I did notice more leaders describing themselves as those who serve churches. That was encouraging.

Yes, yes, I know that the Bible, including the New Testament, uses the term "leader." And yes, I know that followers of those leaders are called to be submissive to them. I know all of these passages and I believe and teach them. But I also believe that our emphasis shows what we most believe and value about leadership, and it isn't Matthew 20. How do we keep missing the vital heart of leadership? Get ready for a shock. We start going amiss by missing the real heart of God, his true nature. And what is that? Servanthood, pure and simple. While he can be described accurately in many ways with many terms, his overriding nature is simply that of a servant.

We know that we are to imitate Christ and we do try to imitate many things about him. But is our natural inclination to gird ourselves with a towel and wash the feet of the unworthy? That was exactly what Jesus did in John 13. He wasn't temporarily lowering himself to make a point; he was acting in accordance with who he was by nature. He was a servant, has always been one and always will be one. Just consider what is being said in Hebrews 7:25. "Therefore he is able to save completely those who come to God through him, because he always lives to intercede for them." Jesus lives to serve you and me, right now and always, twenty-four/seven. Do you always live to serve the people God has given you to serve (lead)? Do they describe you as a great servant, an imitator of Jesus with this most fundamental leadership quality defining you best as a leader?

Agape Love Equals Servanthood

While many words describe Jesus and what a righteous life consists of, he summed it up as love. Loving God with all of our being and loving our neighbor as ourselves are the foundation of the entire Law (Matthew 22:36-40). Paul stated the same principle in slightly different words in Romans 13:8-10. That said, John warned us not to mistake love for a feeling without actions demonstrating that love. 1 John 3:18 says, "Dear children, let us not love with words or speech but with actions and in truth." A similar summation word for me is one I have used quite a lot, the word "surrender." This term encapsulates the words *faith* and *trust.* Actually, faith is used in at least six different, but related, ways in the New Testament, all fitting into the idea of surrender.

One other summation word is what this chapter is about, servanthood. It encompasses all that love is, just like the word surrender encompasses all that faith is. Those terms help me grasp the bottom line and provide the big picture view of the very essence of who God is and who I am to be as I strive to imitate him. The key point of Matthew 20 about the servant/ slave being the greatest of all is illustrated by Christ coming not to be served but to serve and give his life as a ransom for many. I find Luke's parallel account of the same truth striking. Luke 22:25-27: "Jesus said to them, 'The kings of the Gentiles lord it over them; and those who exercise authority over them call themselves Benefactors. ²⁶ But you are not to be like that. Instead, the greatest among you should be like the youngest, and the one who rules like the one who serves. ²⁷ For who is greater, the one who is at the table or the one who serves? Is it not the one who is at the table? But I am among you as one who serves.'"

Perhaps even more striking is what Jesus says in Luke 12 about his return in words very similar to those in his Matthew 25 parable of the ten virgins. In both passages, he is describing our need to be ready and watching for his return. Then Luke 12:37 records this shocking statement: "It will be good for those servants whose master finds them watching when he comes. Truly I tell you, he will dress himself to serve, will have them recline at the table and will come and wait on them." Do you grasp the implications of what he is promising us who remain faithful until he comes again? We, the servants of the most high God will continue being served by the most high God. Christ and the Father are both described in Scripture as Lord of lords and King of kings. They obviously can also be described as Servant of servants. In some inexplicable way, God will still serve us in the world to come as he does now. He is a servant, always and forever. He cannot be otherwise. His nature never changes, nor can it. "Jesus Christ is the same yesterday and today and forever" (Hebrews 13:8). A remarkable truth hidden in plain sight, indeed!

Chapter 9

•

Implications of Matthew 20

Let's go back to the text of Matthew 20:25-28 and ask of it some questions that are begging to be asked. Why did Jesus begin with a description of worldly leadership? That was obviously where the apostles were conceptually. Ten of them were indignant toward James and John. Why? Because the two were being worldly in their thinking and the ten wanted to see them get help? No, not at all. They were envious that the two beat them to the punch in seeking what they perceived to be the ultimate leadership positions as men would see them. Plus, those two had their mother to advocate for them in their request. Position, not servanthood, was the foundation of their thinking and desires regarding leadership. Of course, we would never be like that, would we?

I look with embarrassment back to a time when my family of churches was characterized not simply by worldly leadership concepts, but by military ones. I describe this sad period in Chapter 4 on leadership styles in my book, *Dynamic Leadership*, under the subheading, "The Military Model." I included nineteen examples of the military model, all suggested by leadership groups in several different churches. The suggestions came in rapid-fire order; it didn't take much time to figure it out. Sadly, most of us bought in to accepting parts of the model, although some were better or worse than others. But no one from our earlier days can deny that our leadership was full of worldly concepts and practices. Nor do I think that many today would deny that we have too many vestiges of worldly leadership left in our churches right now. It was once clearly taught that the members should serve the leaders, not vice-versa. Servanthood has not carried the day, which means that we still don't understand the basic nature of God as the Servant of servants.

Another question that arises from these verses is how does Jesus fit in? He was obviously correcting the views of the apostles and calling them to both servanthood and even slavehood in their views of leadership. But he used himself as the ultimate example. He came into the world as a servant and giving his life up on the cross could demonstrate slavehood. Two passages come to mind.

John 15:13

[13] Greater love has no one than this: to lay down one's life for one's friends.

Romans 5:6-8

[6] You see, at just the right time, when we were still powerless, Christ died for the ungodly. [7] Very rarely will anyone die for a righteous person, though for a good person someone might possibly dare to die. [8] But God demonstrates his own love for us in this: While we were still sinners, Christ died for us.

Dying for a friend is servanthood. Dying for one's enemies could be called slavehood. Jesus is the greatest example of both to ever walk the earth, but as old Jim said, Jesus didn't become a servant or slave by virtue of becoming a man. His nature is that and always was. In an article I wrote entitled, "Life's End Game and the Greatest Story Ever Told,"[xi] I describe the plan of the cross as being in the mind of God before he created Adam and Eve. He knew what introducing creatures of choice into the world was going to cost him. He had already filled out the price tag before the merchandise existed. If that doesn't define servanthood, I don't know what would. Always and forever, he does what is best for us, whether we can understand it at the time or not. Some of my greatest gains have come through the times of greatest pain, and my arduous stay in the hospital marked the highlight of this principle. I wrote three health updates on Facebook, and this is the last paragraph of the final one.

> The normal reaction to hearing these details goes something like this: "Goodness, that must have been tough, but I'm so happy you made it through!" That is an appropriate response, to be sure, but mine is different. Yes, it was very challenging and sometimes very scary, but it was the greatest spiritual experience of my life— by far. The spiritual insights I gained were simply marvelous. I knew even in the worst days that if I survived, I would need to start a YouTube channel and share through some form of podcasts what God had taught me. If I could skip the illness episode but also miss the spiritual insights, would I choose that? I don't think so. As crazy as it may sound, I believe I would go through it all again (but only with the help of your prayers) to learn what I learned and to connect to God the way I have. I love and appreciate you more than you imagine. Stay tuned! I will resume my radiation treatments Monday, but only have about 9-10 remaining. No more chemo! Please keep me in your prayers that all of the cancer will be eradicated. God bless you!

Finally, if the greatest quality of a follower of Christ is servanthood, especially for leaders, it has to be the greatest quality with which to define Christ himself. It simply has to be; it must be; it cannot be otherwise. Certainly God is light and love and many other things, but his overriding supreme quality is servanthood to the nth degree with no limitations or boundaries—

up to and including death for his enemies. If that is what I am to imitate, especially if I am a leader, it changes so much about how we see him, ourselves, our roles and our relationship with him. God's greatest description is *Servant*.

Chapter 10

•

God's "Harshness" in the Old Testament

Once I understand intellectually that the supreme description of Jesus is that of a servant, I have to clear out any hurdles that keep me from emotionally accepting this marvelous truth. Since God's "harshness" in the Old Testament has been one of my greatest hurdles to clear, let's just start here. What did God have to work with when he brought the Israelites out of four hundred years of bondage? It wasn't spirituality. They had long forgotten the God known by their ancient ancestors like Abraham and Moses. They were idolators as were their captors and owners. Just how difficult would it be to deal with several million people in that condition? Just imagine taking a million people out of some of the countries today which are immersed in the most extreme form of Muslimism with the intent of leading them into living by true Christian principles. Can you not picture the absolute necessity of dealing with many of them in ways that uninformed observers might call harsh?

Illustrations like that help me understand that whatever God did in Old Testament times was necessary for the good of the majority as history unfolded. God was still a servant seeking the best for his people, but those people left him little choice in applying discipline that he must have hated applying. Even as God meted out judgment, Ezekiel describes his heart. "Say to them, 'As surely as I live, declares the Sovereign LORD, I take no pleasure in the death of the wicked, but rather that they turn from their ways and live. Turn! Turn from your evil ways! Why will you die, people of Israel?'" (Ezekiel 33:11). God is literally begging them to repent and live, but their failure to repent left him no choice.

The capacity for evil in the human heart is difficult to fully grasp. This must be kept in mind as you wrestle with what seems to be amazingly harsh discipline in that Old Testament setting. Jeremiah 17 describes the blessings of the ones who trust in God and put their confidence in him, but also describes the plight of those who do not. What determines the difference? The heart. "The heart is deceitful above all things and beyond cure. Who can understand it? [10] I the LORD search the heart and examine the mind, to reward each person according to their conduct, according to what their deeds deserve" (Jeremiah 17:9-10).

I've always been drawn to a comment by Spock in the old Star Trek series: "The needs of the many outweigh the needs of the few." When God punished individuals in the Old Testament period, at least three things should be kept in mind. One, they deserved it. God is just and the punishment he dished out fit the sin. Two, those punished set an example to hopefully prohibit others from imitating their sinful behavior. Many passages in both the Old Testament and New Testament make this point. "Let us, therefore, make every effort to enter that rest, so that no one will perish by following their example of disobedience" (Hebrews 4:11). 1 Corinthians 10 provides a shockingly specific example of such disobedience and its consequences, and also assures us that Christ was right in the middle of it all. Thankfully, the section ends by assuring us that God can deliver us from temptations that lead to such consequences if we will but trust and follow him. Read it carefully, noting the symbolism involved between this Old Testament setting and our New Testament setting. Being in the church as a baptized, communing member does not guarantee our salvation, that's for sure.

1 Corinthians 10:1-13

[1] For I do not want you to be ignorant of the fact, brothers and sisters, that our ancestors were all under the cloud and that they all passed through the sea. [2] They were all baptized into Moses in the cloud and in the sea. [3] They all ate the same spiritual food [4] and drank the same spiritual drink; for they drank from the spiritual rock that accompanied them, and that rock was Christ. [5] Nevertheless, God was not pleased with most of them; their bodies were scattered in the wilderness.

[6] Now these things occurred as examples to keep us from setting our hearts on evil things as they did. [7] Do not be idolaters, as some of them were; as it is written: "The people sat down to eat and drink and got up to indulge in revelry." [8] We should not commit sexual immorality, as some of them did—and in one day twenty-three thousand of them died. [9] We should not test Christ, as some of them did—and were killed by snakes. [10] And do not grumble, as some of them did—and were killed by the destroying angel.

[11] These things happened to them as examples and were written down as warnings for us, on whom the culmination of the ages has come. [12] So, if you think you are standing firm, be careful that you don't fall! [13] No temptation has overtaken you except what is common to mankind. And God is faithful; he will not let you be tempted beyond what you can bear. But when you are tempted, he will also provide a way out so that you can endure it.

Many of such examples came at times of transition when keeping people on the right path was fundamentally important for their future. One such time was when the church was very young and two people set a bad example that led to them becoming an unexpected but effective type of example for both the church and the community. Read the account of Ananias and Sapphira in Acts 5:1-11. The last verse shows the effectiveness of God taking their lives. "Great fear seized the whole church and all who heard about these events." Verses 13-14 make the point even clearer. "No one else dared join them, even though they were highly regarded by the people. [14] Nevertheless, more and more men and women believed in the Lord and were added to their number."

Three, God directly killing the disobedient or them being killed via the laws of capital punishment didn't necessarily mean that they were lost spiritually. I cannot imagine that Uzzah touching the ark to steady it, through ignorance of the Law's stipulations for carrying the ark, was thereby condemned spiritually. The accounts of this unfortunate situation are found in both 2 Samuel 6 and 1 Chronicles 13. Both accounts should be read to get the complete picture. Further, those being put to death through capital punishment were admonished to repent before being killed. It is not that much different today in America, as clergymen are made available for those on death row. Repentance doesn't always remove the consequences of our sins, but it can remove the sins in God's mercy.

I understand that the above paragraph contains my opinion on the matter. However, that opinion doesn't come simply from my sense of what should be true. Moses gives us an example that clearly illustrates the point I have made. He was God's man and God's hero, and yet he sinned grievously enough that God refused to let him go into the promised land. The description of his sin leaves us questioning the severity of the punishment, but since God is perfect, whatever was involved in this sin was sufficient to warrant the punishment. Was Moses lost spiritually for this sin? Of course not! He and Elijah appeared with Jesus on the Mount of Transfiguration in Matthew 17. God is just but he is merciful. James 2:13 says that mercy triumphs over judgment. God shows mercy in every way possible under the umbrella of justice. Servanthood in action leads to life answers to life questions. Thus, let's ask and answer this question: What are the fruits of servanthood? Coming in the next chapter!

Chapter 11

•

Servanthood and the Abundant Life

Jesus did come to give us life to the full, the abundant life (John 10:10). That is his goal as the greatest servant of all. Satan will try to convince us otherwise, but don't be fooled. God loves us and wants us to be full of joy. If you really believe that to be his goal, you will read the Bible in a way that expects to find that truth. For example, look at this oft-quoted passage: "Then he said to them all: 'Whoever wants to be my disciple must deny themselves and take up their cross daily and follow me. 24 For whoever wants to save their life will lose it, but whoever loses their life for me will save it'" (Luke 9:23-24). To follow Jesus, we must practice self-denial, daily cross-bearing and loss of life. Wow—sound exciting? Without understanding the servanthood of Jesus, these challenges sound demanding and unreasonable. But if you accept that Jesus wants the absolute best for you, the passage reads quite differently.

Let's start with self-denial. It may sound too demanding, but is it? Stop and think about what your selfish self leads to when it is in control. Just about everything bad. Selfishness is a malady that destroys happiness and relationships and a bunch more. Self-centered people are miserable, and they make those around them miserable (if taken seriously). I had two grandmothers who were polar opposites. One was focused on herself, her needs and her problems. The other was always focused on others and their needs. The first was negative and often miserable. The second was positive and always happy. I was around her a lot and never once saw her otherwise. You will never convince me that self-denial is a bad thing. Nor is it a burdensome thing. It frees you up to become more like God and the more you are like him, the happier you will be.

What about taking up a daily cross—it that a negative? Is that a heavy burden? For starters, look at Matthew 11:28-30. "Come to me, all you who are weary and burdened, and I will give you rest. ²⁹ Take my yoke upon you and learn from me, for I am gentle and humble in heart, and you will find rest for your souls. ³⁰ For my yoke is easy and my burden is light." Jesus doesn't say that his burden isn't a part of our lives; he just says that it is a good part, a part that brings rest to our souls. Compared to the burden of selfishness and sin, it is light indeed. Even when we suffer for him, understanding these principles, we will feel blessed to do it. "However, if you suffer as a Christian, do not be ashamed, but praise God that you bear that name" (1 Peter 4:16).

Another very relevant passage in this discussion is Galatians 2:20. "I have been crucified with Christ and I no longer live, but Christ lives in me. The life I now live in the body, I live by faith in the Son of God, who loved me and gave himself for me." Imagine a life controlled by Christ and no longer controlled by our sinful self. He loves us and has proved it by sacrificing himself for us. The Servant of servants is now living in us and leading us. There have been a number of times in my life when I felt like I was a third party watching on, watching myself do things that were pretty amazing. On those occasions, it was so obvious that Jesus was in control, working in me and through me. The feeling I have when this application of Galatians 2:20 becomes reality is simply euphoria. What could be better than being as one with him? Nothing that I have ever found. To be used by God and sense his presence as you are being used has no equal.

The Bible is full of passages that sound demanding but are quite the opposite in their effect.

Acts 20:35

In everything I did, I showed you that by this kind of hard work we must help the weak, remembering the words the Lord Jesus himself said: "It is more blessed to give than to receive."

Luke 6:38

Give, and it will be given to you. A good measure, pressed down, shaken together and running over, will be poured into your lap. For with the measure you use, it will be measured to you.

Philippians 2:3-5

Do nothing out of selfish ambition or vain conceit. Rather, in humility value others above yourselves, [4] not looking to your own interests but each of you to the interests of the others. [5] In your relationships with one another, have the same mindset as Christ Jesus.

This last passage goes on to describe Jesus as a servant, with the end result of him being exalted to the highest place (verse 9). If servanthood is our highest calling, you can be sure that it will carry the highest reward possible. It did for Jesus, and it will for you and me.

I have been amazed at all the ways that Luke 6:38 has been true in my life. You simply cannot outgive God. I think back to a time when I didn't go to church often as a young married man and didn't want to go when I did. I just went to get my new wife off my back! A number of surprising statements were made in sermons by the preacher who eventually became the vessel God used to turn my life around spiritually in ways that I could never have imagined. One of them was when he was preaching about giving to the church financially, a tithe no less, and quoted Matthew 6:21. This verse says simply that where our treasure is our hearts will be also.

He made the point that most people look at this passage backwards, thinking it says that where are hearts are, our treasure will follow. Of course, there is truth to that also. But he said that if we put our treasure in spiritual things, applying it to church contributions, our hearts will follow. In other words, giving our money will change our hearts. I thought this was ridiculous, to be candid, but I decided to start doing what he recommended to just test out one of the many spiritual concepts he was stating as absolute truths. My wife's urging also factored in. She was the only spiritual one in our marriage at the time. Even with a questionable attitude on my part, we started tithing and have never stopped. He was right. Rather, the Bible was right. Luke 6 is also right. I have never in those nearly sixty years since then been able to outgive God, and I have more real-life examples to illustrate that fact than I have time to share. Amazing! Simply amazing!

Chapter 12

•

Servanthood and a Righteous Life

The effects of sin in our lives are always bad and often disastrous. I didn't believe that when I was young. I was taught it by my mother, but I hadn't seen enough evidence yet to buy in to the concept. I had friends and relatives who were doing things that I knew were supposed to be wrong, but it seemed like they were getting by with it. I couldn't yet see the consequences in their lives. That phase didn't last too long. Those who were my age started getting married without God's principles as a guide. Their lives began unraveling in time, and when their children reached adulthood, the picture came into even sharper focus.

Underneath the smiles and Facebook stories, the rigid rod of reality told the true tale. The last line of Fantine's song, *I Dreamed a Dream,* in the famous musical, *Les Miserables,* describes the outcome of many whose lives are not centered on God. "Life has killed the dream I dreamed." That is the present condition of most in our society, leading to frustration and anger which can stay pent-up for only so long. It is being acted out in many, many horrific ways as I write these words. And without Christ in our lives, it will only get worse. The consequences of sin cannot be denied.

Our nation provides a good example of how it gets worse. I remember a conversation with an older friend in Boston years ago who had grown up there. He recalled being in elementary school when the attack on Pearl Harbor occurred. He said that once they got the news, their teacher led the whole class in Bible reading and prayer for the rest of the school day. Can you imagine that happening in a Boston public school classroom today? I remember reading a historical novel about the early settlement of the East Coast of the US, and in very challenging times, it wasn't unusual for the mayor of Boston to call for a fast of even several days to cry out to God for help meeting those challenges. Now we have drifted so far away from the Bible as an accepted standard that we shouldn't be surprised at the consequences of unrighteousness permeating our society. The kingdom of self and self-serving has taken the place of biblical servanthood demonstrated and called for by Jesus.

If sin is the disease, servanthood is the cure. Those focused on serving are already immersed in self-denial. Sin is not nearly the temptation that it is to people who are mainly focused on self or even on merely avoiding sin, and therein lies the failure of the religion of my youth. It was all about avoiding sin, not serving others in the name of Christ. Most who call themselves Christians live about the same as their neighbors, except they avoid outward sins. They are just about as self-centered and materialistic as everyone else. Self-denial is thus defined very narrowly indeed. It is about what not to do rather than being focused on what Jesus did and still would do—and wants to do in and through us. Do you see the difference?

Every follower of Jesus has the responsibility of serving. It is not a burden but a blessing, an opportunity and a privilege. Some followers of his also have the special *gift* of serving (Romans 12:7). Those with the gift serve more gracefully and naturally than the rest of us, and in doing so they provide an example to help the rest of us grow in that area. My wife, Theresa, has this gift in abundance. She lives to serve. She can't help serving. She is compelled. It doesn't matter who we are with or where we are, her gift will come out. It is pretty amazing to watch and sometimes a bit embarrassing for me to watch. She will take over situations involving total strangers as she tries to serve them. In restaurants, I've seen her serving strangers by arranging chairs and tables and holding babies and doing whatever she thought would help them have the best time. They seemed to sense her gift and were quite relaxed about it all, appearing to view her as a part of their family on a temporary basis. As I said, it's amazing to watch.

When we began recording the first episodes of my podcast series, I talked to Theresa about how I wanted things to function. I explained that the recording sessions weren't about us entertaining fellow Christians or focusing on hospitality. It was business and we had to stay both quiet and focused. So, said I, let's just put bottled water in the refrigerator and inform them to serve themselves as needed. She listened very attentively and seemed like she understood exactly what I was saying and why, and agreed to follow the guidelines I suggested. But as Rick, my technology friend, and I were setting up all the equipment prior to the arrival of the guests who were to be in the podcast, I glanced over at our dining room table. Of course there were bottles of water there, along with pumpkin bread, pumpkin chocolate chip cookies and a huge bowl of fruit salad and the sauce with which to top it. In earlier years, that might have led to an argument, but I didn't say anything negative to her. She can't help it. She has the gift of service. Servanthood should have been her middle name!

Theresa is, not surprisingly, one of the most spiritual people I know. When we are focused on serving others, we are not focused on self and thus sin's temptations have much less effect on us. Sometimes when we are praying together and confessing our sins, I find myself wishing that all I had to confess was what she did. I have "big boy" sins; she has "little girl" sins—all because she is a far better servant than I am. As I was thinking about this servanthood concept recently, it occurred to me that I should ask her a question that I'm not sure I have asked her directly before.

I understand the challenges of male lust, which I have shared about honestly in describing my own battles, something that any honest man will admit can be a problem. But I wondered what the challenge of that sin might look like for her. The results of a fairly in-depth discussion were about as expected. She just doesn't struggle with it, and I believe her because I know her. Servants focus on the needs of others, not the *bodies* of others. Jesus was around women all of the time, women who adored him, and yet he never lusted once. Regarding my wife, we are talking about a woman who has loved the sexual part of our marriage. Sex has been a big part of our marriage but her having lust for other men has not. The ramifications of being a servant are wide and deep. Spiritual righteousness and servanthood are inseparably connected and the more you think about it, the more you understand why.

Chapter 13

•

Servanthood and Awareness Awakened

Servanthood brings an increased awareness of many types. Having an awareness of the situations faced by others and their subsequent needs is an obvious one. The awareness of our own nature, complete with its weaknesses and sins is another. It has been pointed out that awareness in Western culture is highly individualistic whereas in Eastern culture, it is more of a group awareness. Western culture has spawned the "me" generation concept. When it is all about me, selfishness in its many forms chokes out servanthood. Even our choice of "causes" to get involved in often carries a self-focus with it, for our choices may be based mainly on what makes us feel good about ourselves. Thus, involvement in causes doesn't necessarily equate with being servants. This is why being self-aware spiritually is absolutely essential.

True servants are increasingly aware of their own shortcomings and sins. While in the hospital, becoming more and more aware of God's supreme nature being that of servanthood, I was also becoming more and more aware of my lack of a servant spirit. During one of my sleepless nights, I had a thought jump into my mind seemingly out of nowhere. It involved me and my wife and my electronic preferences, phones in particular. The story has a necessary back-story to fully appreciate what I am about to describe.

I officially decided to become computerized in 1992. I was writing quite a lot even back then, but without a computer. I had an assistant whose tasks included typing out my hand-written material on his computer. He kept telling me that writing on a computer was fundamentally important, not just in terms of saving both of us time, but in terms of what he described as something like thinking through your fingers. He finally convinced me to give up my computer phobia and buy one.

At that time, I knew just enough about computers to know that there were two basic types: Macintosh and Windows. I had no idea what the differences were, and which might be best for me, so I started asking advice of my computer using friends. One thing became obvious quickly. The Apple folks were not only sold on their products but sold to the point of sounding arrogant and even cultish. Purely because of that response, I decided to go with a Windows based computer. I reasoned that I had enough pride already and didn't need to join the Apple cult to worsen it. Seriously, that was the true back-story behind my initial choice.

The problem I didn't see coming, or see once it came, was that in my resistance to all things Apple, I had developed the same problem in reverse. I became a Windows snob, often deriding Apple products. Then came smartphones, with Apple being the leading innovator in this new field. I became very thankful very quickly when Android phones made their appearance. I didn't have to use an iPhone! Yea! I had a choice and I made it. Since that first Android phone, I have owned many, and I was always quick to tell my iPhone friends that Android was the superior system.

Now we come to the real issue that God brought to my attention while in a hospital bed contemplating death and him and all points in-between. My wife is not technology oriented and initially showed no interest in smartphones, Apple or Android. Phones were used to make phone calls. End of story—until the grandchildren had smartphones and wanted to exchange texts with their grandmother. Knowing that the grandchildren had iPhones and that they were supposedly more user friendly, I bought my wife one of those dreaded iPhones. That initial purchase was now over a decade ago.

Since that time, I have been impatient and unhelpful with Theresa in the use of her phone. I didn't want to figure out anything about it, meaning that I wasn't willing to serve her by learning how it functioned. Adding insult to injury, I often spoke disparagingly of her phone when she was having a problem with it. *I. Was. Not. A. Servant!* Not only did I fail to serve, but I was impatient and critical when she needed help with her phone. And this attitude and treatment was aimed at the most wonderful wife in the world, the one whom I love and cherish! What a servant husband would have done is switch to an iPhone when his wife first got one in order to help her with the unavoidable learning curve involved.

This whole story flooded my mind and heart in a flash, all at once, on that fateful night in the hospital. The next day, I shared the story not only with Theresa, but with my son Bryan's whole family. They knew my attitudes and had heard my complaints and sarcasm directed at iPhones, and they all needed to hear me repent. Then they needed to see my repentance in action. I asked Joy to order two new iPhones, the latest and greatest of them at the time, which she did. Now my wife and I both have iPhone 13 Pro Max phones. I can and do help her with her phone now. I should have done this long ago—and would have if I had been imitating the God whom I love. He didn't just change something he owned to serve us; he changed himself into a human being and died for us—unimaginable servanthood!

I remember an old song, very popular in its day, *You Always Hurt the One You Love.* The first few phrases are heart-breaking, but true. Why do we hurt the ones we love? They are about the only ones who love us enough to put up with it. Sad thought, that. I wish that my little phone story was the only such memory I have about ways I have hurt my wife, failing to be the servant that God has called me to be. I imagine that this one story is enough to get the wheels of your memory turning, and hopefully enough to help you repent also in whatever area comes to mind (and heart). In my case, Theresa had a hard time believing that I was serious about really repenting. It took seeing my tears of repentance to grasp how deeply grieved I was over my sins of selfishness and pride.

My hospital insights about the nature of God led to my insights about the nature of Gordon—and to repentance. I'm just so grateful to God for revealing both types of insights to me during my time of sitting on the brink of eternity with him. I needed to be there, and his servant heart was moved to take me there. Spiritual insights are found in the package of God's nature that we humans can never fully open, but try we must, and try with fervor, determination and consistency. Let's do it!

Curiosity being what it is, some of you are wondering how I am faring with my iPhone. For a while, I remember still preferring Androids for some technical reasons, but now I have no idea why and don't care. The iPhone is fine and is serving me well and helping me to serve Theresa with hers. Just so you know, I also bought an Apple computer years ago and used it daily and exclusively for six months. It was a good computer, but not as suited to my particular uses as is a PC. But no more disparaging talk about brands of computers or phones. They are all good and simply matters of preference, just like brands of a myriad of other products. My iPhone and I are doing well in developing our relationship, as my wife and I continue to do in deepening ours (after 59 years of marriage). Repentance is sweet and an integral part of servanthood for us humans!

Chapter 14

•

Servanthood and the
Multiplication of Influence

Through the years, I have had many leaders in many settings. I only remember details about two types and two types only: those who were harsh and those who were servants. Both types have led me to pray a lot. The former caused me to pray for patience and forgiveness and for them to repent and change or be taken out of leadership roles. The latter caused me to offer many prayers of thanksgiving. Many prayers of the latter type continued—long after I was under their leadership, even after their deaths in some cases. (I think especially of Wyndham Shaw. Chapters 3 and 4 in my book, *The Power of Spiritual Relationships*[xii] will demonstrate why.)

Between the harsh ones and the servant ones were the majority whose leadership I experienced, but I don't remember too much about them. I suspect that they were focused on themselves enough to keep me from being so. You will be remembered by those whom you hurt or serve, but by few others. When you reach old age, if you are fortunate enough to live that long, you will think about your legacy, what you are leaving behind of yourself in the hearts and lives of others. Do something about it now by imitating God in being a servant.

In speaking about basic human needs, or love languages, acts of service are always included in the list. It happens to be my primary love language. I thank God for those who have served me and are serving me now. At the top of my prayer list, a long list, is my request for God to bless those who have prayed for me to be cured of cancer and who prayed for God to spare my life while I was in the hospital sitting with God on the brink of eternity. I can't keep from shedding tears when I think about those in this category. Why? Because they are servants—they served me.

I imagine that some, perhaps many, who knew of my serious illness were never moved to pray at all. But I know for a fact that large numbers of my friends prayed earnestly and frequently for my healing, and still pray for me. I wrote this part originally near the beginning of September 2022, and then the jury was still out on whether my cancer was cured or not. Due to the severe reaction to the chemotherapy medication, I only took a partial amount of it. After getting out of the hospital, the radiation treatments resumed. I trusted that God had heard enough prayers from his servants, who were also my servants, to let that suffice for a cure.

After the radiation treatments were finished, I had to wait three months for further testing since the radiation continues to work for three months after treatments end. On September 19 (oddly, my father's death date and my brother-in-law's birthdate), I went back to the surgeon who found the cancer the second time and when I awoke from the anesthesia, she informed me that she took no tissue samples because there was nothing there to take. Exactly two weeks later, the radiation oncologist said in our virtual appointment that the MRI scan taken a week earlier was perfectly clear, so she would see me a year from then for another scan. The surgeon insisted on doing a check every three months, at least for the first year, which she did. To be honest, it didn't sink in quickly. The early diagnosis which turned out to be a false/negative made it harder to believe. What was quickly and easily believed is that the huge number of prayers for my healing by my spiritual family all over the world made all the difference. I will never be able to thank them enough. There are no words…

We all have the basic human need of being accepted; thus, we fear rejection. We want to be approved, to be included, to be considered important, hopefully even essential to those with whom we associate. Do you not think that servanthood will gain these rewards, and far more? We don't serve to be served in return or give in order to be given to, for serving is its own reward. It is more blessed to give than to receive. Considering others more important than ourselves brings benefits far beyond what we might expect. Jesus changed the world by being the world's greatest servant. You can change your world by being the best servant you can be, with God through the Holy Spirit enabling you to keep growing in this capacity.

Our Greatest Influence

Selfishness is natural; selflessness is unnatural. Yet, as with most things, what comes naturally is of the world and what takes genuine effort and self-denial is of God. Trust him that his way, *the Via Dolorosa,* is the path to glory. It will change you, and better, it will change others. Influence is about helping others rather than impressing others, which makes true leadership one of servanthood, from beginning to end. Trust Jesus enough to trust that fundamental truth.

The greatest influence you can possibly have on another's life is helping them become followers of Jesus. If becoming a Christian, coming into a saved relationship with God through Christ, is our first priority, guess what? We should feel compelled to see that as a starting place in being a servant to others, helping them find that same saved relationship. Although I didn't attend the Summit Conference in Orlando mentioned earlier, I did watch a lot of it virtually. The very first class I watched addressed the topic of raising up the next generation.

All three presenters approached the subject in somewhat different, but complementary ways. One spoke about campus ministry and what they were doing in his city. He didn't speak about what they *ought* to be doing; he spoke about what they *were* doing and had been doing recently. He had two impressive younger generation disciples speak as a part of his presentation. It was all so convicting. It reminded me of why I was attracted to my family of churches in the first place. I saw back then the majority of our membership in action, having a determination to imitate the mission of Jesus, "to seek and save the lost" (Luke 19:10). As we seek to influence and serve others in every way possible as we strive to imitate Jesus, let's not forget what our first priority with others should always be—helping them know Jesus.

Chapter 15

•

Surrender's Spectrum

I've written much about servanthood, but servanthood is predicated upon a faith that can be described as surrender, letting go and letting God take control. The second book I wrote was *The Victory of Surrender*. Although written long ago, it has remained the "crowd favorite." As I have continued to wrestle with my view of God and the nature of my relationship with him, an important truth has dawned on me. Surrender falls on a spectrum with at least three positions. We often speak of people being on "the spectrum," meaning the spectrum of autism. There is a wide range encompassing the condition we call autism. Similarly, there is a range on the spectrum of spiritual surrender. All surrender is beneficial, but not all surrender is equal. My recent insights have shown me that my own past concept of surrender was not at the pinnacle of the spectrum. Where we are on that spectrum is tied inseparably to our conception of the nature of our God.

At the low end of the spectrum is what I would describe as resignation, simply resigning ourselves to any given situation that we find challenging. Even non-Christians adopt this approach to challenges when they can find no other, as I mentioned briefly back in Chapter 2 . But for them, God is not in the equation. As Christians, we accept such resignation as ultimately being from the hand of God, whether we feel good about it or not, whether we are really trusting Romans 8:28 or not. Even if God is working all things together for good, what we are experiencing doesn't seem good and trusting it will turn out for our good can be an elusive goal indeed.

I remember hearing a sermon over a half century ago that used the term "resign" in three ways when speaking about finding ourselves in challenging situations. The preacher said that we could resign or quit, just give up—application number one. Or we could just resign ourselves to the objectionable situation, grin and bear it or grit our teeth and bear it—application number two. Or we could re-sign, sign back up for another go at handling the problems facing us with grace, God's grace—application number three.

Merely resigning ourselves to what we see as a negative situation may have some spiritual convictions behind it, but the level of trust is not impressive. Thomas the apostle seemed to operate with this level of surrender, as these passages indicate.

John 11:16

Then Thomas (also known as Didymus) said to the rest of the disciples, "Let us also go, that we may die with him."

John 20:24-29

[24] Now Thomas (also known as Didymus), one of the Twelve, was not with the disciples when Jesus came. [25] So the other disciples told him, "We have seen the Lord!" But he said to them, "Unless I see the nail marks in his hands and put my finger where the nails were, and put my hand into his side, I will not believe."

[26] A week later his disciples were in the house again, and Thomas was with them. Though the doors were locked, Jesus came and stood among them and said, "Peace be with you!" [27] Then he said to Thomas, "Put your finger here; see my hands. Reach out your hand and put it into my side. Stop doubting and believe."

[28] Thomas said to him, "My Lord and my God!" [29] Then Jesus told him, "Because you have seen me, you have believed; blessed are those who have not seen and yet have believed."

Thomas is called "Doubting Thomas" for good reason. He always followed Jesus despite his doubts, but his trust was clearly at a low level. Thus, his surrender was not the kind to inspire others. Like all the apostles, I believe the reality of a resurrected Lord ultimately changed him and he became an inspiration. None of the apostles were stellar examples of believers in the resurrection until after they had seen a resurrected Jesus. But despite their difficulties in believing throughout Jesus' ministry that he was going to die and be resurrected, they still had the commitment to follow him no matter what. Resignation, even accompanied with doubts, still falls on the surrender spectrum, if we simply keep following.

Level Two

The second level on the surrender spectrum is when our primary focus on Jesus is that he is the Lord, the Master, and we are his servants. Such is a biblical analogy to be sure. Consider Luke 17:10: "So you also, when you have done everything you were told to do, should say, 'We are unworthy servants; we have only done our duty.'" As with all passages, context is extremely important. In Luke 17, Jesus had just given them a shocking lesson about forgiveness. It should be unlimited, said he. In their shock, they exclaimed, "Increase our faith!" After telling them that even a small amount of faith, the size of a mustard seed, could accomplish great things, he focused on the need for them to simply keep obeying as servants.

They had a long way to go yet in developing faith, and obedience was the path to follow in developing it. They would reach that third level of surrender, as we will see, but they were not there yet. We sing the old hymn admonishing us to "trust and obey," but sometimes we have to obey in order to develop trust. Mark 1:15 suggests this principle in these words of John the Baptist: "Repent and believe the good news!" John 8:31-32 is similar, when Jesus said that fully grasping truth and being freed by it follows obedience ("holding to his teaching"). In this passage, initial belief has to move on to obedience if we are to be made free of Satan's hold on us through our surrender. I have a plaque hanging on the wall of my office that says, "It is easier to act yourself into a better way of feeling than to feel yourself into a better way of acting." Meditate on that one, for it directly ties into the obedience/faith principle.

I think this level of surrender was what motivated me to write my book on the subject. Surrender has always been one of my biggest challenges. I think that is true for most of us, but not all of us. I have known a few who lived in level three. No matter what happened to them, they simply trusted that God was in control and the principle of Romans 8:28 was inevitably going to be proved true. Wilner Cornerly was one such disciple. When we moved to Phoenix in 2003, the financial challenges in a time of church upheaval were such that the role for which he was hired simply wasn't feasible financially. Joe Silipo and I took Wilner out to lunch, and with as much sensitivity as possible, fired him. Joe and I were both crying as we did it. Wilner was calm and simply unflappable, full of trust in God and the plans God had for his life.

He ended up going to Chicago to be a part of a ministry staff there, and those who hired him later thanked us for firing him! A few years afterwards, he developed terminal cancer. I was invited to speak in his congregation in Chicago when he was nearing his end. Despite his pain, he was present for one of the last staff meetings he ever attended. With two of us by his side helping to hold him up, he led the closing prayer. His attitude about having cancer and facing death were the same as when we had the job termination talk. God is God and all is well. What a hero of the faith! What an inspiration! What an example of surrender at the very top of the spectrum!

I think my book described both levels two and three. We often start off at level two and end up at level three. Truthfully, I often write much better than I think, feel and live. That could be seen as hypocrisy, but in this case, I don't think it is. As one old preacher of yesteryear said, "I don't have any respect for any preacher who doesn't preach better than he lives, but neither do I have any respect for any preacher who isn't trying his best to live as well as he preaches." I like that. I like to think that's me. I believe it is. I am not nearly all that I want to be for God, but I want it badly and I'm striving for it and will until I draw my last breath. I believe I have fought to reach level two of surrender many, many times in my life when challenges came fast and furious. When I gave it my best to simply trust and obey, or obey and trust, I yielded to Jesus as my Lord and Master and ultimately found peace. That peace at the end of the process was either level three or very close to it. However, level three is, as I said earlier, inseparably tied to our view of God and his nature.

Level Three as a Progression

So, what is level three on the surrender spectrum? It is what Jesus was leading his twelve disciples to, as described in John 15:15. "I no longer call you servants, because a servant does not know his master's business. Instead, I have called you friends, for everything that I learned from my Father I have made known to you." The apostles started at level one, progressed to level two and finally reached level three. Seeing yourself as a friend of God will motivate in ways that seeing yourself merely as a servant to the ultimate Master will never accomplish.

I think of my earthly father in this connection. When he was younger and quite a force of nature, I was afraid of him. I did what he said out of fear. When he was old and becoming feeble, my motivation wasn't fear at all, but desire to do anything to serve him and nothing to disappoint him. Love and quality of relationship had replaced fear. I think of level three surrender as a combination of warm love and total trust of a loving Abba. I often picture it in the words of Psalm 131:1-2. "My heart is not proud, LORD, my eyes are not haughty; I do not concern myself with great matters or things too wonderful for me. ² But I have calmed and quieted myself, I am like a weaned child with its mother; like a weaned child I am content."

I think that is where I am with God now. Like I was with my earthly father when he was old, I am not afraid of God. 1 John 4:18-19 tells us that we shouldn't be and why. "There is no fear in love. But perfect love drives out fear, because fear has to do with punishment. The one who fears is not made perfect in love. ¹⁹ We love because he first loved us." I just don't want to disappoint him in any way. He has been so amazingly kind to me. His kindness has led me to repentance time and time again, as he intended (Romans 2:4). His kindness toward me is almost impossible to conceive. From birth until now at age 81, he has blessed me beyond measure, almost beyond comprehension. As the old song puts it, I stand amazed in his presence. I stand amazed at all that he has done in my life, the ways that he has orchestrated it, inserting just the right people and the right situations into it—at just the right times.

I am a blessed man who has lived a blessed life, from birth to death, whenever and however death may come. I cannot imagine how or why he has blessed me so. I sometimes attribute it to having married my little angel of a wife, Theresa, and reasoned that since God is determined to bless her, I was able to come along for the ride by being one with her in marriage. That does make some sense, doesn't it? But then I look at my early years, my BT (before Theresa) years, and even though spirituality was neither a fact nor an interest, he blessed me anyway—repeatedly. Unbelievable! What a God I have—a

Father, an Abba, a Friend!

Only when these three terms seem real to us in our relationship to God will surrender level three become a reality. I am not there all the time, but I want to be. I was there during my 23-day hospital stay, sitting with God on the brink of eternity. When I left the hospital, I was in a euphoric state. It wasn't because I was finally being discharged from a very challenging period, although I was thankful to be going home—alive. It was because something happened in those long nights as I sat with God, my Friend, and contemplated eternity. As I stated earlier, I don't know just how to describe what happened to me emotionally and spiritually. When I was in what could have been mistaken for a manic state, as Tom Jones thought, it no doubt seemed like it. Tom wasn't far off in his observations about that part. It was an unbelievable experience. Euphoric for sure.

I wish I could say that it lasted until this present moment, but it didn't. Like many emotional highs, we do come back down to reality. Anyone who has attended an inspirational conference knows what I am talking about. Even Jesus coming down from his experience on the Mount of Transfiguration knows what I am talking about. But in spite of the descent back into the real world, the hospital stay was one of my life's greatest adventures. I was born wired for adventures. I love them. I need them. God has provided them all of my life. Even some of the greatest challenges I have faced have proved to be great adventures as I look back on them.

My tendency to imagine worst case scenarios hasn't stopped God from giving me best case scenarios. I stand amazed in his presence. I stand blessed in his presence. I stand grateful, exceedingly grateful, in his presence. He is the Servant of all servants, and he has served me for a lifetime. O God, my Abba, my Friend, help me to imitate you in becoming a servant, growing more and more into your likeness as I represent you as your image bearer, striving to demonstrate you as the greatest Servant of all times and all worlds!

Chapter 16

•

A Sobering Reality in a Night to Remember

As I shared one part of my hospital story with my friend Otoma Edje via email, he made this comment: "What you share about 'getting your house in order' is very sobering." It is also connected with servanthood, as you will deduce. Early in my hospital stay, as I've said, I was in bad enough shape that the possibility of dying was almost constantly on my mind. For that reason, I asked my son, his wife and three sons to come to the hospital, together with my wife, on one of the first nights I was there. My oldest grandson was about to turn 24 and my youngest about to turn 17. They were old enough to be a part of the serious discussion I had in mind. Discussing death is to some morbid, but to me it is simply reality, howbeit a sobering one. I shared my concerns that I might die and shared my concerns that I hadn't done all I had intended to fully set my house in order. I began sharing what those latter concerns were.

I had two file cabinets full of old documents, most of which were irrelevant and unneeded. I explained which of them would be relevant if I died and asked them to have the rest shredded. I also explained that I had a closet and desk drawers full of electronic items that would need to be disposed of as well and how to best do that. I then moved on to how to help Theresa with the immediate finances, although the long-range issues were in a document that I've kept updated for years on my computer.

Periodically, I have given Theresa paper copies to keep in a safe place, since she isn't much of a computer person.

In trying to describe the short-range issues, I asked Bryce, my oldest grandson, who happens to be a business graduate with a financial job, to get a pen and paper and start making notes. As I attempted to recall needed usernames and passwords, I tried to verify their accuracy on my phone. Being in somewhat of a hallucinatory state, the phone screen looked weird, as if someone had put a totally different operating system on it. I could not figure out how to make passwords work on it. That was a frustrating experience. But I went on to share as many details as I could think of in my altered mental state about what to do in the event of my death.

Some of my family members were crying as they seriously contemplated my possible imminent death, and some were concentrating on what I was trying to explain. Knowing it was a strange night, I told them that I had been trying to teach them how to live well but also wanted to teach them how to die well. Dealing with the realities involved is, and was then, sobering. It was a night none of us will ever forget, but at the end of it, I felt good about it.

Since I didn't die, my house is now in much better order. Six boxes of documents in file folders and other materials have been professionally shredded. My old buddy from Boston, Rich Evans, flew in for several days to help me with the electronic collection of now useless (to me) items. He dealt with five old computers, three electronic tablets and two phones. Hitting the delete button doesn't fully delete files, but Rich knew how to erase it all. With some of the equipment left, he thought of ways it could be used by others; some obsolete items we simply threw away; and the remainder we dropped off at a recycling center.

I updated my "In the event of my death…" document with all sorts of instructions in it, including those for my memorial service, and gave Theresa a printed copy. Of course, I have an updated will in a safety deposit box. (I hope you have one too—everyone should.) I feel relieved to have all of that accomplished, for when I do "fly away," my family members will find it much easier to deal with the details. I spoke with a widow friend shortly after her husband died, and she just shook her head and said that he had been a "clutterbug." I don't want to be remembered with any such term! Nor do I want to leave my family with the clutter to dig through and deal with as my deceased friend did.

Many people have asked me how Theresa handled all of this, knowing that her husband might well die. Two words come to mind: maturity and spirituality. Theresa took it a day at a time and never came close to freaking out. That's just not her. Her response to a conversation I shared with her years ago provides a good insight into how she processes the reality of death. One of my great friends during our Phoenix years was Jerry Jones, and along with his wife, Karen, we were very good friends as couples. Jerry and I served as elders for some years after the initial appointment of elders in the church in which we were members.

Jerry was a classic disciple of Jesus, although he was converted later in life. He had such a soft heart, but such a courageous heart. We faced some tough times during several years when the church was going through a seriously challenging time. Jerry was a rare bird as a leader. I taught repeatedly and insistently that as leaders, we couldn't let concerns about reactions and responses determine the decisions we made and the paths we chose, but only what was right for the church and righteous before God. Jerry in response was all in, like few leaders are capable of being, conflict avoidance and sentimentality being what they are. I couldn't have made it through those tough years without him.

His view of death was beautiful. Once when I was with him and his wonderful wife on a trip to serve in an orphanage just over the Arizona border in Mexico, he asked me a question. He said something to this effect, "Given our ages, you and Theresa do talk about what to do when one of you croaks, don't you?" I burst out laughing at his terminology and when I later shared it with Theresa, she just cackled. After that, she bought him birthday cards with pictures of frogs on the front and the inside captions saying in some form, "Glad you haven't croaked yet!" But he did croak. He was in the hospital on dialysis when he decided it was his time. He opted to come home to die and did within a few days. The last time I called to speak to him, Karen said that he was asleep and had only brief periods of being lucid when awake, but promised that if he had another such period, she would call. He did and she did. Jerry and I had such a wonderful talk and he encouraged me greatly. He died the next day. I was blessed to speak at his memorial on the one-year anniversary of his death. I was his teacher, but he taught me about dying well, a lesson that I want to pass on to others. I can assure you that Jerry was quite ready to croak. His house was in order. Is yours?

Chapter 17

•

Our Dual Existence

Aside from those who supposedly have multiple personalities, all of us are two people in one. My favorite passage in the Bible, 2 Corinthians 4:16-18 makes our dual nature clear and also defines what our focus should be in light of that nature. "Therefore we do not lose heart. Though outwardly we are wasting away, yet inwardly we are being renewed day by day. [17] For our light and momentary troubles are achieving for us an eternal glory that far outweighs them all. [18] So we fix our eyes not on what is seen, but on what is unseen, since what is seen is temporary, but what is unseen is eternal." Although the terminology of "wasting away" isn't exactly pleasant to contemplate, over time its truth becomes more and more obvious. That said, the next part about daily inward renewal should motivate us to make sure we are doing just that. Spending quiet times with God isn't just a nice idea; it should be seen as an absolute necessity.

We have an outward part and an inward part, the latter being made in the image of God. I recently told someone that I still felt like I was 35, although my body reminded me that I am 81. Why do we feel like that as we age, still young in spite of our aches and pains and wrinkles? Our inner person, our soul or spirit, doesn't age. It doesn't even sleep nor need sleep—that's why you dream all night. The real you, the inner person, doesn't need sleep and has been created for eternity. Death, biblically defined, is simply the departure of the spirit from the physical house it lived in, the body.

James recognizes this distinction in James 2:26. "As the body without the spirit is dead, so faith without deeds is dead." Paul put it this way in 2 Corinthians 5:1-4: "For we know that if the earthly tent we live in is destroyed, we have a building from God, an eternal house in heaven, not built by human hands. [2] Meanwhile we groan, longing to be clothed instead with our heavenly dwelling, [3] because when we are clothed, we will not be found naked. [4] For while we are in this tent, we groan and are burdened, because we do not wish to be unclothed but to be clothed instead with our heavenly dwelling, so that what is mortal may be swallowed up by life." Peter continues with the tent analogy in 2 Peter 1:13-14 thusly: I think it is right to refresh your memory as long as I live in the tent of this body, [14] because I know that I will soon put it aside, as our Lord Jesus Christ has made clear to me." Tents are temporary dwelling places and thus provide an apt analogy to describe life in a physical body.

During the early part of my hospital stay, as mentioned, I was both hallucinatory and delusional at times. However, when people started talking to me, I somehow escaped that condition and reentered reality. And trust me, many people talked to me. Since I was in a teaching hospital, medical students came in frequently to interview me. Given my condition, I was shocked that that would even be allowed. But I gave it my best effort and answered their questions and added some advice. I was also shocked that I was able to engage in a coherent way and make sense in those conversations and in many others with medical personnel.

One of my specialists, Dr. Fuller, came by often to speak with me, sometimes spending up to a half hour at a time discussing my condition and possible steps forward. My case was both very unusual and somewhat complicated. Yet, he allowed me to help make several decisions that were not in line with normal protocol, and which carried some risks. That example alone confirms that I was having a mild form of what could be called an "out of body" experience in that my inner part was still functional despite the condition of my physical part. He trusted my reasoning in those cases enough to let it influence his own thinking. Not all doctors listen well to their patients, but the best ones trust that we know our bodies well enough to at least contribute to the cumulative data about them.

The fact that I was able to do that, repeatedly, attests to the truth that we are in fact dual beings. My inner person was able to engage when my outer person was extremely sick. Quite an interesting experience, and a surprising one to me, but it shouldn't have been. I am two people in one, and the part of me made in the image of my Father isn't nearly as dependent on the other part as might be assumed. That was a cool discovery. While one part of me was deathly ill, the other part was capable of rising above that illness and carrying on almost as normal. Interesting—and impressive! We are indeed fearfully and wonderfully made, as Psalm 139:14 says.

The biggest takeaway from this insight should be to help us make sure our primary focus in life is clearly on the spiritual side of it. Spiritual trainwrecks are likely results when this is not the case. Usually, the older we become, the greater the challenges. I have seen too many older people lose their way spiritually by not being able to handle those challenges, but it doesn't have to happen like that. Continuing to grow spiritually by nourishing our inner person is the antidote. Don't let your focus shift to the temporary; keep it on the eternal. Paul said it best in 2 Corinthians 4:18 in these words: "So we fix our eyes not on what is seen, but on what is unseen, since what is seen is temporary, but what is unseen is eternal."

Chapter 18

•

Servanthood and Perspectives About Salvation

Jesus' primary purpose in his earthly ministry was made clear in passages like Luke 19:10, "For the Son of Man came to seek and to save the lost." The last thing he said to his apostles before ascending back to heaven further demonstrated this purpose. "Therefore go and make disciples of all nations, baptizing them in the name of the Father and of the Son and of the Holy Spirit, [20] and teaching them to obey everything I have commanded you. And surely I am with you always, to the very end of the age" (Matthew 28:19-20). Meeting as many strangers as I did during my hospital stay made me wonder how many were in a right place with God spiritually. I want to have the same purpose Jesus had in helping people come to a saving faith in him, the ultimate act of servanthood.

The next to last book I wrote was also the shortest I've ever written, entitled, *God, Are We Good?*[xiii] What prompted me to write the book is the awareness that most of my neighbors and extended family members know little Bible. What they think they know most often has not come from their personal study but from what others have said, which boils down to personal opinions. Thus, opinions are shared and used as a substitute for biblical knowledge, which is a dangerous situation. Jesus is quite clear in Matthew 7:13-14 that most humans are not going to heaven. But how many people are even aware of this passage? Few. Hence, the motivation to write that book. I have given and sent copies to friends, family members and neighbors in the hope that they will read and learn some of the most basic, yet most serious, teachings of the Bible about salvation. Ignorance does not remove responsibility and accountability before God.

How Do We Get Saved Spiritually?

The Bible is crystal clear about the necessary commitment to Christ and his way of life. The level of commitment Jesus described in passages like Luke 9:23-26 and Luke 14:25-33 is not negotiable; without it people are lost. Anyone not committed to producing the fruit of the Spirit (Galatians 5:22-24) but is rather producing the acts of the sinful nature (Galatians 5:19-21) cannot be saved. These latter verses leave no doubt about the matter. "[19] The acts of the flesh are obvious: sexual immorality, impurity and debauchery; [20] idolatry and witchcraft; hatred, discord, jealousy, fits of rage, selfish ambition, dissensions, factions [21] and envy; drunkenness, orgies, and the like. I warn you, as I did before, that those who live like this will not inherit the kingdom of God."

In addition to the commitment to following Jesus as a lifestyle, a highly important question is how we get saved spiritually in the first place? To me, the biblical examples in Acts, the history of the establishment and spread of the original church, provides a model for us to follow today. The later letters to the churches align quite well with those examples. Yet, most of the Christian delineated churches don't teach the plan of salvation the same way I believe the Bible teaches it. That is a mystery to me. I just don't understand why this is the case, and yet it is. My understanding of the conversion process is that it includes baptism as a part of a faith response. Most teach that baptism is not a part of that process, but rather is an outward sign of an inward grace, an act following conversion and not a part of it.

Read the following passages I quoted in my little book and see what you think. The first of these is from the first gospel sermon preached after the resurrection by Peter to several thousand Jewish people in Jerusalem. The examples following this are accounts of the conversion of individuals—an Ethiopian official; a Gentile jailor in Philippi; and the apostle Paul.

Acts 2:36-38

"Therefore let all Israel be assured of this: God has made this Jesus, whom you crucified, both Lord and Messiah." [37] When the people heard this, they were cut to the heart and said to Peter and the other apostles, "Brothers, what shall we do?" [38] Peter replied, "Repent and be baptized, every one of you, in the name of Jesus Christ for the forgiveness of your sins. And you will receive the gift of the Holy Spirit.

Acts 8:34-38

The eunuch asked Philip, "Tell me, please, who is the prophet talking about, himself or someone else?" [35] Then Philip began with that very passage of Scripture and told him the good news about Jesus. [36] As they traveled along the road, they came to some water and the eunuch said, "Look, here is water. What can stand in the way of my being baptized?"

[38] And he gave orders to stop the chariot. Then both Philip and the eunuch went down into the water and Philip baptized him.

Acts 16:29-34

The jailer called for lights, rushed in and fell trembling before Paul and Silas. [30] He then brought them out and asked, "Sirs, what must I do to be saved?" [31] They replied, "Believe in the Lord Jesus, and you will be saved—you and your household." [32] Then they spoke the word of the Lord to him and to all the others in his house. [33] At that hour of the night the jailer took them and washed their wounds; then immediately he and all his household were baptized. [34] The jailer brought them into his house and set a meal before them; he was filled with joy because he had come to believe in God—he and his whole household.

Acts 22:14-16

"Then he said: 'The God of our ancestors has chosen you to know his will and to see the Righteous One and to hear words from his mouth. [15] You will be his witness to all people of what you have seen and heard. [16] And now what are you waiting for? Get up, be baptized and wash your sins away, calling on his name.'

Other passages from Acts could be included in this list, and others could be added from the epistles written to the early churches. I will just include a couple of the latter.

Romans 6:3-5

Or don't you know that all of us who were baptized into Christ Jesus were baptized into his death? [4] We were therefore buried with him through baptism into death in order that, just as Christ was raised from the dead through the glory of the Father, we too may live a new life. [5] For if we have been united with him in a death like his, we will certainly also be united with him in a resurrection like his.

1 Peter 3:21

And this water symbolizes baptism that now saves you also—not the removal of dirt from the body but the pledge of a clear conscience toward God. It saves you by the resurrection of Jesus Christ.

Yet, My Tensions Remain

As I wrote my little book, I became more aware of

a tension I often feel in my own historical perspectives regarding salvation. My background in what is often called the "Restoration Movement" exposed me to churches that were decidedly doctrinally oriented. The "Reformation Movement" (Protestantism) focused more on *reforming* the existing church of the 1500's (Catholicism) rather than *restoring* the original church, but the latter is an understandable and reasonable goal. Yet in time, Restoration churches became so doctrinally focused that nothing was more important than getting our doctrines right and in total alignment with what the Scriptures taught— or what we thought they taught. My present family of churches had its roots in the Restoration fellowship, and thus we too have maintained a significant focus on doctrinal correctness.

My tensions enter when I see the biblical commitment being lived out by those whose conversion experience doesn't line up with the Bible as I understand it. For example, my hospital experience demonstrated that more people than I might have imagined are serious about Christ. Erin, one of the sisters in my local church group, had a large banner printed up to encourage me and then took it to a marriage retreat being taught by my old friends, Roger and Marcia Lamb. Many attending signed the banner and most of them wrote short but encouraging notes on it. Joy brought the banner to my hospital room and taped it in a location so that anyone who entered my room saw it almost immediately.

The Perfect Banner for Sharing

This prompted many conversations and opportunities for me to share my faith. I was surprised and encouraged by the number of medical workers and students who seriously engaged in spiritual discussions with me. The last medical students who came in to interview me as a patient were refreshing. One of them, a young woman, said that she was a part of the campus ministry in the medical school and had just returned from a mission to South Texas. As they were getting ready to leave, she asked if we could pray together. Several others had done the same during my stay. She held both of my hands and led one of the most spiritual prayers I had heard in a long time.

In our short time together, we didn't discuss theological issues. This was neither the time nor the place. I did tell many people about my website, and many of them promised to look it up. Plenty of articles are found on it which cover both theological and practical spiritual issues of all types. The probability is that most of the people whom I encountered in that setting have a different view of the conversion process than I do. What about them? How would God answer them if they asked the question posed by the title of my book, *God, Are We Good?* Therein lies my tension, how to view the combination of commitment to Christ and doctrinal accuracy (or lack thereof), especially involving such an important topic as conversion.

A conversation some years ago with an older leader was helpful to me in this regard. In his profession, most of those in his professional setting (Christian college professors) were professed Christians, and many of them were serious about their commitment to Christ. My friend said that he felt more in common with many of them than with some of those with whom he attended church on Sundays. The latter ones may have shared his same theological beliefs, but their lives didn't compare favorably to many of those in his professional association. Although a very conservative person doctrinally, he made the statement that he had hope for those whose doctrine regarding salvation differed from his, but he didn't feel that he could give them hope. In other words, he couldn't assure them that they were good with God. Yet, he believed that they most likely were. I have quoted him many times, for I feel much the same. I will always teach exactly what I believe the Bible says on any matter, but only God is the Judge. He will do what is right and it might not be exactly what we expect.

PS—An Unusual Book Ending

In my short book, I dedicated a chapter to my tensions just described, but I also dedicated a following chapter to the tensions I would feel if I were on the other side of the issue. After finishing the manuscript for that book, I added a closing section I termed a "Postscript." A postscript is something you think of later and add, which is exactly what I did sometime after I finished writing the book. I will include some pertinent quotes and observations from that postscript.

> Broadly speaking, sin is breaking God's laws in our personal life and in holding and/or teaching erroneous doctrinal beliefs. Life and doctrine are both important (1 Timothy 4:16), and they may be compared to the wings of an airplane. A plane cannot fly without two wings, and our lives cannot please God without life and doctrine aligned with what he commands. Are both equally important?
>
> But here is my question in closing: is forgiveness of both types of sins (life and doctrine) available in equal measure? We know and teach that God's grace toward our personal life sins is exceedingly broad. When you consider that through sins of commission, we sin by our words, our actions, our thoughts, our motives; and through sins of omission, by what we leave undone, it is simply overwhelming to contemplate. Yet, we teach and preach that God will forgive us through the blood of Christ for all of it if we claim Jesus as Lord and have strong intentions to please him, with the direction of our lives demonstrating those intentions.
>
> Moving over to the sins of a doctrinal or theological nature, are we now in a different arena, where God's grace is no longer quite so amazing? We base our hope for heaven not on our performance, but on God's grace, a grace that shapes our desires

to please him and determines the direction of our lives. Thus, his mercy shows itself in our lives as desire and direction rather than as performance and perfection. Will his grace motivating that same desire and direction be sufficient to overcome sins of a theological doctrinal nature? If not, why not?

I closed the book by quoting 1 John 2:1-2 where we are assured that Jesus died for the sins of the whole world and then ended with these final comments.

Are those sins of the whole world only life sins and not theological sins? All I can say in closing is that I am a sinner and in need of abundant mercy, and am thus quite content to leave the ultimate judgment to God about who is right with him and who is not. I can do no more and no less than strive with all my heart to follow his teachings with both my life and my doctrine and urge others to do the same. Thankfully, God will take it from there.

When I meet and spend time with spiritually minded people, regardless of their doctrinal beliefs, I feel a close kinship with them. I focus on the fundamentals of what it means to be a Christ follower and rejoice in our shared commitment. If we are able to spend enough time together, I will get around to discussing doctrines and doctrinal differences, but I don't start there and don't make that my major focus. I also will introduce them to my website and ask them to scan through the article titles, read some of them and communicate with me about that experience. But I am not their Judge and I'm not going to act like I am. I am thankful and encouraged to interact with anyone who loves my Jesus.

Chapter 19

•

But—It's Still a Narrow Road

I have already said quite a lot in this series about how highly Jesus valued the quality and practice of servanthood. The next chapter after this one is dedicated to the hospital staff who served me in amazing and often challenging ways—all with a smile! But does servanthood alone ensure that we will be with God in eternity? In other words, are there other roads to heaven besides the one Jesus established, which we call Christianity? Let me add for clarification that I am referring to biblical Christianity, not American Christianity (and there are many differences). Like the last episode, answering such questions tugs at the heart in ways that make even approaching the subject emotionally difficult. But let's continue to examine all that Jesus meant by the road to heaven being a narrow one.

Having covered my somewhat conflicted views regarding seriously committed spiritual people who have a differing view of conversion than I do, I still do not question Matthew 7. Before we read this passage, let me mention my concerns for my relatives, neighbors and friends that led to the writing of "God, Are We Good?" What I have found in the older generations is not only a lack of Bible knowledge, but an amazing trust in human opinions about the topic of salvation. Attending funerals, memorials, celebrations of life, or any other end-of-life service is often quite alarming to me. If I believed the speakers at those types of services, I would have to conclude that virtually everyone must be going to heaven when they die. But is that what the Bible teaches? Let's answer that question by taking what I call the "funeral test." This test is based on Matthew 7:13-14, 21.

Matthew 7:13-14, 21

"Enter through the narrow gate. For wide is the gate and broad is the road that leads to destruction, and many enter through it. [14] But small is the gate and narrow the road that leads to life, and only a few find it... [21] "Not everyone who says to me, 'Lord, Lord,' will enter the kingdom of heaven, but only the one who does the will of my Father who is in heaven.

Now honestly, what do you get from reading those verses? Isn't it obvious that most people will end up in hell and few in heaven, and further, that claiming to be a Christian doesn't make you one? In our day of biblical illiteracy, most people are totally unaware of what Jesus clearly said in passages like this one. They just share opinions, and guess what? The one called the great deceiver and the father of lies, Satan himself, has done his job amazingly (and sadly) all too well. The vast majority of people, including many whom I know and love, are among the deceived. They don't come close to living the life Jesus is calling us to live, and yet they feel spiritually safe in their condition. If they don't know what the Bible actually says, why would they not?

Memorial services alone would provide them with the feeling of safety. They hear that everyone is safe in the arms of Jesus, in a better place and now at home with God and all of their dearly departed loved ones. It is simply heartbreaking to me. That is why I wrote that little book a few years ago. That is why I try to share with everyone I can, urging them to study the Bible, with me or others who know what it teaches about salvation. I urge them to ask the question posed in the book title, "God, are we good?" and then to study and seek biblical answers to the question.

While in the hospital conversing with many, many hospital workers, I realized that a significant percentage of them didn't come from a Christian perspective to begin with. In their associations with those who claim a Christian perspective, they hear little to nothing about Jesus being the only way to salvation. In our modern post-Christian setting, the assumption even by those claiming Christianity as their religion, is that every "good" person is going to be just fine after they die. But what does the Bible say? Here are a couple of verses to consider.

John 14:6

Jesus answered, "I am the way and the truth and the life. No one comes to the Father except through me.

Acts 4:12

Salvation is found in no one else, for there is no other name under heaven given to mankind by which we must be saved."

Those verses are not hard to understand, are they? All roads don't lead to heaven; all religions don't lead to heaven. I appreciate every person who is trying hard to be good, and who are good in comparison to many other humans, but from a spiritual perspective, none are good enough to be saved without the blood of Christ. Romans 3:10 says there is no one righteous in and of themselves, and two verses later it says that none are good. We may appear both good and righteous compared to many other people, but when compared to Jesus whom we are to imitate, the picture is quite different. No wonder Romans 3:23 sums it up in these words: "for all have sinned and fall short of the glory of God." Christ must be accepted on his terms as the Lord of our lives. He cannot be our Savior without also being our Lord (Master). Verses could be multiplied to demonstrate this truth. Luke 6:46 puts it this way: "Why do you call me, 'Lord, Lord,' and do not do what I say?"

Acts 17:22-31 makes the point quite clear that religions outside Christianity are not acceptable to God. Here is Paul's conclusion as he spoke to the people of Athens who practiced idol religions of many kinds. "In the past God overlooked such ignorance, but now he commands all people everywhere to repent. [31] For he has set a day when he will judge the world with justice by the man he has appointed. He has given proof of this to everyone by raising him from the dead" (Acts 17:30-31). During the Mosaic period, non-Jews were not judged as strictly as after Christ came and established the New Covenant. But now Christ is the solution to the problem of sin and will be the standard by which all will be judged.

In the next chapter, I am going to express my profound gratitude for the care I received from medical workers, most of whom are amazing servants. My appreciation for their service knows no bounds, but it doesn't blind me to the realities of sin and righteousness and the basis of salvation. When Jesus encountered the Rich Young Ruler and called him to a standard he wasn't willing to accept, it did not negate the love Jesus had for him. Mark 10:21 says that Jesus looked at him and loved him, but then he gave him the Lordship challenge which was rejected. I'm sure this hurt the heart of Jesus, but God's standards for being saved cannot and will not be compromised by him. Will you compromise them? That's the question I am asking here. I simply cannot and I pray that you will not.

Thus, while I can commend a serious commitment to Jesus and the Bible, I cannot commend a watered-down version of Christianity nor an adherence to another religion besides that of Christ. The road is narrow that leads to salvation and I am always going to point people in every feasible way to seek that narrow road. Are you? If we truly believe the Bible, we don't have any other option. Sharing our faith and pointing people to the Bible is the Christian's only alternative. I want to have this heart and the life which reflects that truth. I want to imitate Paul's heart when he spoke to King Agrippa. "Then Agrippa said to Paul, "Do you think that in such a short time you can persuade me to be a Christian?" [29] Paul replied, "Short time or long—I pray to God that not only you but all who are listening to me today may become what I am, except for these chains" (Acts 26:28-29). May God give us the convictions and the heart of Paul!

Chapter 20

•

Medical Workers Are Servants

One of the medical workers who often served me during those long nights in the hospital had a genuine spiritual interest, and that led us to several spiritual conversations. He was a deep thinker and the concept of our purpose in this life was one topic he wanted to discuss. I had already come to my firm conclusion that God's basic nature is best understood as Servant of servants, not only as Lord of lords and King of kings. The latter two are more about his sovereign authority, whereas the first is about his heart and nature. With that in mind, it dawned on me that life's broad purpose is to begin by getting right with God and then representing him by being the best servant possible to the most people possible. That's the essence of our purpose on planet earth—to be God's image bearers as we imitate Jesus after becoming his spiritual child. In doing this, we just need to figure out the giftset with which God has blessed us and use it to the full.

Healthcare workers are servants, many of them amazingly so. I have always felt that way, for I have had many friends and family members who served in these roles. Since the Covid pandemic hit in early 2020, most of us have elevated our views of medical professionals to hero status. The NFL season of that year was played in front of empty stands for the most part. Weird. However, at the Super Bowl held in Tampa in early 2021, many vaccinated medical workers had been invited and were in attendance. When that was announced and the cameras turned to show them, I couldn't keep from crying. I can't now. Why? Because of their courage to put their lives at risk to serve people like me.

Joy, our daughter by marriage, is a Pediatric RN. Many of the mothers coming in to give birth during 2020 had Covid and she cared for them and their beautiful newborn babies. There were shifts without many babies being born and at times she was assigned to work in the emergency room. She spent hours in the presence of those battling the virus, fighting for their lives. Joy, and many like her, braved the circumstances and did their jobs. They were, and are, my heroes. They are praiseworthy servants.

Some medical workers perform tasks that you don't ordinarily even stop to think about. When I went into the hospital, I was too weak to do nearly anything. I was rolled in with a wheelchair and helped from that into my bed. I literally could not lift my heels off the bed. And guess what? I couldn't get up to go to the bathroom either, even though I had severe diarrhea and was throwing up in projectile fashion. I had my diaper changed by more different people in that hospital than when I was a baby (by far). But they did it with a great attitude. When I apologized for causing them to have to clean me up, they replied cheerfully that this was why they were there—it was a part of their job. As sick as I was, the process wasn't really awkward or embarrassing. I couldn't help being in my condition and my heroes were there to help me. Thankfully, I could at least talk and thank them profusely for their service. May God bless those who serve in ways that I would find very difficult.

The hospital I was in has a major focus on serving cheerfully. The surveys they send out repeatedly asked about our experiences with medical personnel and the attitudes with which they served us. I've never been in a more upbeat, happy atmosphere medical setting. It was an atmosphere of servanthood with a smile and I've no doubt that my healing was significantly assisted by that type of service. I have wished for some way to thank them after the fact. I even considered going back up to that twelfth floor and trying to find certain ones to again thank when back in a state of sound mind and body. The next section describes interviews medical students had with me and some of the advice I gave them, which included this very topic.

Advice From a Patient

The University of Texas Southwestern Medical School is a part of the sprawling campus which houses the hospital I was in for those 23 days. As stated previously, it is the largest medical school in Texas, which is impressive given the size of the state and the number of medical schools in the state. It is also nationally well known for many reasons. Thus, the hospital I was in is known as a teaching hospital. In the earliest and worst days of my stay there, I was surprised by the entrance of a professor in the school along with several of her students. She explained that a part of their schoolwork was interviewing patients. Although it made sense to me, I was in such bad shape that I couldn't imagine the teacher subjecting me to that experience. However, I decided to make the best of the opportunity and hope I made sense in so doing.

One of my first topics to share with them was the importance of keeping positive, upbeat attitudes in working with patients. I shared the results of studies I had read about, showing that medical personnel affected their patients significantly just by their attitudes. I recalled one study involving a hospital with two floors of patients having serious heart problems, life threatening ones in fact. One floor was blessed with an abundance of happy helpers and the other was not. The death rate on the floor without cheerful workers was alarmingly higher than the mortality rate on the other floor.

Of course, these students were having this very point drilled into them, for that is a vital part of the goal of the school. Mark Mancini, who strongly encouraged me to go to UT Southwestern, said that the doctors made you feel like you were their only patient. I saw a lot of different specialists during my time there, and the majority of them gave off that vibe, making you feel like you were indeed very important to them. I recall one doctor, after she was replaced on my case, who spent some serious time researching my condition and its cause and came back to share her findings with me—in spite of having been reassigned to other patients. Her empathy was clearly genuine as she spoke gently while patting my arm.

Another two pieces of advice I gave to those first students who interviewed me grew out of my own experiences. Both have to do with preventive issues, how to avoid getting sick in the first place by taking care of your God-given body. One of these issues I am convinced helped save my life. Many decades ago, I started having prayer walks early in the mornings. I found that praying while walking allowed me to concentrate better than any other approach. During the early part of the pandemic, I started walking in the afternoons simply for exercise and to reduce the boredom of isolation. That being the case, I found myself walking further and faster than normal. Three miles was a short walk, and four to five became the norm. One day as I neared my house, I looked at my pedometer and discovered I was almost at the seven-mile mark. I continued walking all around my yard until I hit the seven miles.

When I had the extreme reaction to the chemo that nearly killed me, I would imagine that few 79-year-olds have the physical conditioning that I did. I doubt that many in that age group would have survived what I survived, and a definite part of it was being in such good physical condition. Certainly, the multitude of people all over the world praying for me was a huge part of my survival, but I have no doubt that a part of God answering those prayers was my good health prior to the illness. Although the Bible is not a book on how to maintain good health, Paul does make this statement in 1 Timothy 4:8: "For physical training is of some value, but godliness has value for all things, holding promise for both the present life and the life to come."

Some people foolishly almost worship physical conditioning and healthy practices and fail to worship God. No matter how healthy we are and the extent to which we go to be healthy, we still get old and die (if we are fortunate enough to get old first). But since God gives us life in a body, we should take care of it and I'm thankful I have. It made a difference. Although my physical weakness after being discharged from the hospital was significant and lasted a significant length of time, I pushed myself hard to get my strength and stamina back, and it paid dividends once again.

The second part of the preventative advice I gave was about eating. The Old Testament does specify what could be eaten during the Mosaic period and what should be avoided. I am not certain how much of it directly pertained to health, but I am sure that some of it did. I am blessed with a wife who is very health conscious and as a result, considers what we eat to be a very important matter. I am not a picky eater, and that being true, I am fine with whatever she cooks. Most of the fruit and veggies are organic and she simply does not eat red meat. I eat it occasionally when we dine out, but for the most part, I eat chicken, fish and vegetables and try to avoid starches and sweets. I have a challenge with the latter, but I do well enough to avoid developing sugar related physical maladies. I remember having lunch with a brother who said he had just read an article claiming that sugar was seventeen times more addictive than cocaine. I had a hard time believing it, so he pulled out his iPad and showed me the article. There it was, in cyber black and white! I think of refined sugar as a type of poison to help me avoid it.

One of the things that makes Covid more dangerous is being overweight. What makes you overweight? Besides eating too much, eating the wrong things, starches and sweets heading the list. One of my doctor friends in Boston started doing research on what might help him with some of his physical challenges and those of his wife, who had Lupus. He basically discovered that eating meat (including fish and chicken) and vegetables was the most beneficial diet. That is what someone abandoned in a wilderness setting would end up eating. When his patients with Type 2 diabetes followed this way of eating, he was able to take many of them off insulin.

After talking to his wife about their approach, I tried it for one full year—in 2000. I did not eat sweets or starches (bread, pasta, potatoes, etc.). I lost weight without trying and felt better than I had felt in years. My energy level was amazing, and I slept much better than normal. Sad to say, I went off that eating regimen in 2001 and gained back most of my weight. Oddly, I abandoned that eating regimen because I kept losing weight without trying. I thought I might have undisclosed cancer, so I started experimenting with eating what I had avoided for a year. That was a bad choice, but for the last several years, I am back much closer to that same approach, which is a part of my overall good health at the age of (gasp!) 81.

I understand that medical professionals cannot dictate what their patients eat; they can only advise. But I wish they could be more demanding. When Theresa was pregnant with our now 56-year-old son, her doctor was an interesting guy regarding weight control. He set a limit on how much an expectant mother could gain, and if she exceeded it, he dropped her as a patient. I doubt that a doctor could do that today without ending up in court, but if doctors could insist that their patients eat healthy diets, it would be a blessing to them.

Anyway, I didn't go into all of this detail with those students interviewing me, but I did stress the importance of making diet and exercise recommendations (strong ones) a part of their work with patients. I am thankful for my exercise regimen, which helped me overcome the aftermath of my unusual illness episode, and I am thankful for my wife who helps me to be more aware of healthy eating. Both have helped me survive and now return to the health I previously enjoyed before my cancer saga and chemotherapy reaction saga. The oncologist said that regaining my full health conditioning by walking far and fast was unusual for a man my age. My cancer is in full remission mode for now and I feel very good for an *octogenarian*. I am content with that as I try to simply live in day-tight compartments.

Chapter 21

•

Relationships Are All That Matter

I have taught for a very long time that the Bible is all about relationships: relationship with God; with physical family; with spiritual family; and with those who need to become a part of our spiritual family. Those who major in all of these relationship categories are blessed and happy people. The number of friends they end up with is often quite amazing. In my case, it is beyond amazing. I literally have friends all over the world, many of whom would be categorized as dear personal friends, the majority as my spiritual children. But even those in the latter category are viewed in individualized ways. When I went into the hospital, my family didn't want me to be left alone at night. It started with Joy saying that there was no way she was leaving me by myself, so she was staying with me that first night (and did). She stayed other nights as well.

Then Theresa started asking me about possible people who could stay with me during the nights. Everyone she mentioned was a good friend, but I said yes to some suggestions and no to others. The main difference in my answers was a matter involving communication. I didn't want anyone to stay with me who would feel compelled to talk, to keep conversation flowing. I didn't want anyone who would make me feel like I was expected to talk. I was not only "out of it" much of the time, but I had a tube going down my nose to my stomach removing bile. It hurt all the time, but it hurt the most when I was talking. Trying to maintain any kind of a normal conversational setting was beyond me. I needed friends like Job had, at least for the first seven days of their visit with him. During that time, they literally didn't say a word. After that, it all went downhill—badly.

One person came without being asked. He heard about my condition and got on a plane. That was my old and dear friend, then the CEO of HOPE *Worldwide,* Dave Malutinok. He stayed several of the first nights with me and did HOPE work during the days. Of course, I had some conversation with all of those who stayed with me, but we kept it at a minimum. Dave has been a part of my movement of churches for decades and a part of my life for nearly as long. We met in Boston in 1988 and at Wyndham Shaw's request, we began a discipling relationship with Dave and Peggy. A few months later when their second son was born and I visited them at the hospital, I was shocked to be told that their newborn son was named Scott Gordon. Our relationship had a short history at that point, but obviously an important one. That occasion suggested the depth to which our relationship would develop.

Late one night in the hospital, Dave described a concept that hit me as extremely important and quite profound about our church movement. I think I recall being in sort of a fog at the time and asked him to repeat the concept. I immediately said that this should be written into a book and added that helping make that happen was reason enough alone for me to survive my ordeal. I did and we are planning on working on his writing together. It was his idea, and it will be his material, but I plan to assist in any way that I as a writer can. Fog or no fog, that conversation was neither a hallucination nor a delusion. I will never forget it. His ideas in print will help explain not only the real foundation of our movement, but the various actions and reactions of those in our group as well as those outside it, including those who have left it.

Another early overnight visiting friend was Mike Isenberg. I have known Mike from the early days of the DFW Church when he and his wife were on the ministry staff. After nearly two decades serving in this capacity, both he and his wife went back to school to prepare for careers in the medical field. His wife is a specialty nurse, and he is a PA (Physician Assistant). I occasionally call Mike to get some input about medical issues and if he is unable to answer at the time, he immediately finds a way to text, informing me when he will call back. He is a special friend. I asked him why he wanted to stay with me in the hospital, sleep on a sofa and get interrupted at all hours of the night. He said that he felt that God had directly put it on his heart. The combination of his medical knowledge and personal friendship made him a very special overnight guest for me. In any medical consideration, Mike is always very helpful and reassuring.

Although I wasn't receiving any visitors outside family members during the days, a number of other people offered to come and stay the nights. Others wanted to but for one reason or another, simply couldn't. God bless them for their willingness to serve. The others who stayed with me during those long and nearly sleepless nights were family members. Curt Clemens, Theresa's brother (and my brother from another mother), stayed a couple of nights, even though he lived in a different city several hours drive from Dallas. He is a talker, but he worked hard on not talking more than I was comfortable with. I've known him since he was a little kid, and in his youth, he lived with us twice. He is as much family as you can get, that's for sure.

Bryce Gordon, our oldest grandson, works near the hospital and came by to see me many days after he got off work. He spent one night with me, a night which began in the late afternoon. I was just starting to feel well enough to watch TV and since both of us Gordons are sports fans, we watched our Boston teams play (the Bruins and the Celtics) and two other games of each type (basketball and hockey). It was truly a sports night and a fun night despite my condition. Bryce is mature beyond his 26 years, an "old soul" type, according to his dad—my son, Bryan. He definitely sees through the immaturity and fallacies embraced by so many in his age category—thankfully! Anyway, that was a memorable and much appreciated night.

Joy stayed with me several nights and also wanted to be present during daytimes when specialist physicians came to update me on my status. As an experienced nurse, she had questions to ask that were important. Joy's biological father left her family in her youth, although she was able to reconnect with him shortly before he died. He and her stepdad died within a short time of each other, emotional blows to be sure. But I am her dad and she is my daughter. We usually say that she is our daughter by marriage, rather than daughter-in-law, but even that description doesn't explain our relationship. The mother of our niece's husband calls our niece her "daughter-in-love." That works too. Joy is our daughter, just as much as her husband is our son. Relationships are much more heart-connections than biological connections. I'm the only dad that Joy has left, but I am her daddy—heart and soul.

Finally, Theresa ended up staying a few nights with me after my health improved. We will have been married 60 years this coming January 30th. Our love has deepened into something difficult to describe. We are around each other almost every day, all day, and we wouldn't have it any other way. We are comfortable to the nth degree with each other, but it goes far deeper than that. We are still deeply in love, carrying with us the memories of the occasion that started our love affair way back in the fall of 1960. That initial spark of romance is still alive and well, deepened immeasurably by the many decades together since. In those hospital nights, our special indescribable bond made our time together a very special and treasured memory for both of us. It was marriage at its deepest level in one of our toughest times.

Bryan and his family came often to encourage me, and their presence gave me motivation to fight for life and for a return to health. Bryan was especially sensitive about driving Theresa to and from the hospital after dark, since she isn't comfortable driving in traffic at night. Relationships are indeed all that matters, and being on your potential deathbed will remove any doubts about the accuracy of that statement. Study after study has demonstrated that the happiest, healthiest people are the ones with the largest number of positive relationships. In my case, healthy relationships were more than healthy—they were spiritual relationships. I've no doubt that my physical and spiritual relationships made it possible to come back from being on the brink of eternity to survival and ultimately, to a return to health. I'll be back on that brink at another time, and when that comes, my relationship with God will be the one that matters most as I leave planet earth. During my hospital ordeal (and blessing), relationships with family, physical and spiritual, made all the difference. God has been and will be there in the middle of it all. Amen!

Chapter 22

•

God's Love of Variety

I am simply awestruck with God's creation. When we were at our cottage in the countryside of East Texas, I had my quiet times journaling on my laptop, sitting on the porch with the lake across the street in full view. That is what I saw. But what I heard were birds, lots and lots of birds. I remember receiving a call from a dear friend, Walter Parrish (now deceased), while sitting outside on the porch journaling on my computer. He asked where I was at the time. He said it sounded like I was in some kind of bird sanctuary. He was hearing slightly what I was hearing loudly. I also was enjoying a hummingbird who was taking advantage of the sugar water in our hummingbird feeders just a few feet from where I was sitting. Occasionally, one little guy would come towards me and just hover while watching me from about two feet away. God's creation is wonderful and absolutely amazing. He obviously loves diversity, since he created it as he did.

Speaking of diversity, here are a few interesting facts showing just how diverse God's creation really is. Although determining the total number of species of living organisms on earth is a challenge and the estimates vary widely among scientists, over two million species have been identified and described. However, total estimates of the true number of species varies. The most widely cited estimate is 8.7 million species, but many believe there are far more than that. Since we were just speaking about birds, know that there are more than 11,000 bird species that have been identified. Estimates of dog breeds are between 195 and 500. Cat breeds are harder to distinguish, but the experts in that field vary between 40 and 70 in their estimates.

But then we get into the big numbers. Scientists estimate that the total number of fish species in the world is approximately 33,600 and more than 3,000 species of snakes exist on the planet. Scientists believe that there are about 435,000 unique land plant species on earth, with tree species numbering 73,300. In the world, some 900 thousand different kinds of living insects are known, by far the largest group within the various types of God's creatures. That's almost a billion—nearly impossible to grasp. Even more impossible to fathom are the varieties of colors. It has been determined by experts who study such things that there are somewhere around 18 decillion varieties of colors available for your viewing pleasure. That's an 18 followed by 33 zeros. Many more facts and figures could be included here, but you get the point—God is the Creator of unfathomable amounts of diversity, showing his obvious love for it.

United Nations?

Why am I including this topic in writing primarily about insights I gained from a challenging three weeks in the hospital? I had scores of different medical caretakers during those seemingly endless days and nights. The diversity among them was a bit shocking at first and certainly fascinating. From a racial or ethnic standpoint, it was like entering a meeting of the United Nations. I met people whose countries of family origin numbered in the dozens. As we talked, I found that many of them were second generation and had never been to the country from which their parents came. Since I had been to most of those countries, it was exciting to describe them and my experiences there. As would be expected, the physical characteristics of those serving me varied greatly, including their various shades of color. Some had very light skin and some had very dark skin. The majority fell into categories that we would call "people of color." All of them were caring, sensitive, serving human beings, made in the image of a God who loves diversity.

To be very candid, being served by them caused me to think about those of my country who have views that in one way or another could be classified as White superiority or White supremacy. They might not tout it or even realize it, but these thinking patterns are embedded somewhere in their psyche. Such views of one's fellow human beings, realized or unrealized, is a devaluing of other people created in God's image that I have grown to disdain. The concept of White superiority in any form is not only indicative of gross ignorance, it is an affront to God as Creator. It is also the result, as I said, of incredible ignorance.

In the first place, the word "race" itself is a misnomer. There is no such thing as race as most think of it from either scientific or biblical viewpoints. Regarding the scientific viewpoint, I wrote an article several years ago explaining why people are different colors. Although I am not a scientist nor an expert in the field of racial origins, the facts are quite available for anyone willing to do some research. And many of these facts are not recent ones. A well-known anthropologist, Ashley Montagu, who in the same year I was born (1942) published a book entitled, *Man's Most Dangerous Myth: The Fallacy of Race*. This stuck with me not only because the book was written in my birth year, but Ashley was my mother's maiden name. Further, the topic of the book was absolutely intriguing to me. Montagu was quite the interesting character, a Jewish atheist, who surprisingly didn't subscribe to Darwin's views on race (as described in his writings during the latter half of the 1800's).

Darwin believed that Black people were much less evolved than White people, and as a result, less intelligent. Darwin also believed something similar about females generally, regardless of color. But Ashley rejected that part of Darwinism, and along with Albert Einstein, spoke out strongly against the views and ill treatment of Black Americans by White Americans. A part of that action no doubt came from their common Jewish backgrounds and the racism they had endured personally. But it was far more than that to Montagu – it was a matter of science. His views ended up carrying the day with his fellow anthropologists in rejecting any supposed scientific basis for race. Experts in that field by and large agree with Montagu's conclusion that race is a fallacy.

Sunlight and Vitamins

Most living organisms have an incredible capacity to adapt to their environment. Humans obviously share that adaptability. My good friend James Williams, a Black brother in our church, spent his entire career teaching Social Studies to 8th grade students in his home state of Mississippi. He has said to me a number of times that our skin color and other physical characteristics trace directly back to the proximity of our ancient ancestors to the equator. The closer they were to the equator, the darker their skin. Not only is that a simple answer, it is absolutely accurate. But why is it accurate? Primarily it is an issue of sunlight and vitamins, of two types.

The melanin in the outer layer of our skin worked over long time periods to allow one type to be absorbed into the body and the other type to avoid being taken out of the body. Vitamin D must be absorbed in sufficient amounts to build calcium. In northern climates where the sunlight is less available, the skin must remain lighter in tone to make sure that enough vitamin D is absorbed. The other vitamin, called folate, a vitamin B complex, is significantly affected by the ultraviolet light from the sun, and dispersed from the body rather quickly if the skin is light. The body's folate reserves can be reduced significantly in a brief period of time if the sunlight is intense, and the skin is very light in tone. Hence, those in the tropics must have darker skin and the melanin takes care of that. Bottom line, if your ancient ancestors lived in low sunlight areas, they developed light skin; if they lived in high sunlight areas, they developed dark skin. You can read the details and find the information sources in my article on my blogsite, "blacktaxandwhitebenefits.com."

I also have a segment in that article showing that DNA suggests nothing of the presence of different biological races. I read an interesting article online from Harvard's Graduate School of Arts of Science website. It was written April 17, 2017, by Vivian Chou and entitled, "How Science and Genetics are Reshaping the Race Debate of the 21st Century." Under the subheading, "New findings in genetics tear down old ideas about race," the following statement was made: "Ultimately, there is so much ambiguity between the races, and so much variation within them, that two people of European descent may be more genetically similar to an Asian person than they are to each other." What Montague wrote eight decades ago as an anthropologist aligns perfectly with what geneticists are saying right now. Race is a fallacy.

The Bible and Human Nature

From a biblical standpoint, Acts 17:26 could not be clearer: "From one man he made all the nations, that they should inhabit the whole earth; and he marked out their appointed times in history and the boundaries of their lands." Although the earth's one solitary race, the human race, began with Adam,

Noah and his family of eight people were the progenitors of all to follow them, as Genesis 10:32 states: "These are the clans of Noah's sons, according to their lines of descent, within their nations. From these the nations spread out over the earth after the flood." Bible believers need to start accepting what their Bibles say, namely that we are all of one race. If we accept that obvious truth, then we will learn to not only accept our human differences but to rejoice in them. The multitude of different cultures and ethnicities contribute so much value to those of other cultures and ethnicities. Think food, clothes, music, dances, inventions—and the list could go on. In our global age, societies in virtually all nations have more of a mixture in them than most would imagine. Why not admit it, embrace it and enjoy it? It is an undeniable fact—and an irreversible fact.

My own country, the United States, is more wacked out on racial issues than one can imagine. The political quagmire we are in presently has contributed greatly to the problem. While I deeply regret what is happening in our society, I am not at all surprised by it. In my fairly lengthy article on this topic mentioned above, I have this subtitle for one section: "Haters Gonna Hate!" Without Christ and a commitment to imitate him and thus follow his principles, hating is inevitable. It always has been. "At one time we too were foolish, disobedient, deceived and enslaved by all kinds of passions and pleasures. We lived in malice and envy, being hated and hating one another" (Titus 3:3). What Paul wrote two millennia ago describes our present age perfectly, as do more lengthy passages like Romans 1:18-32. I have another long article on one of my two websites asking the question of whether Covid-19 is a discipline of God or not, and in it, I go through the Romans 1 passage in some detail. The world is the world is the world, and without Christ, it always will be.

Why? Easy answer. "We know that we are children of God,

and that the whole world is under the control of the evil one" (1 John 5:19). As children of God, followers of Christ, how do we avoid Satan's control? Once again, easy answer, but challenging to apply given the effectiveness of Satan's deception. "Do not love the world or anything in the world. If anyone loves the world, love for the Father is not in them. 16 For everything in the world—the lust of the flesh, the lust of the eyes, and the pride of life—comes not from the Father but from the world. 17 The world and its desires pass away, but whoever does the will of God lives forever."

One evidence of loving the world is found in a rejection of the beauty of God's diverse creation, especially the human part of his creation. Any view, however subtle, found in our heart of hearts, that places a higher value on one skin color over another is Satanic. It cannot be godly no matter how impressively it might be explained. Knowing enough about how racism of all types works and how it makes people of color feel, I cannot see any evidence of White superiority attitudes without it breaking my heart. Such attitudes are an afront to God and call into question his very design of us human beings as his image bearers. God is love; Satan is hate. Where do you fall on that scale in your views of your fellow humans? Thus, you have my perspective on racism developed even more intensely from a hospital bed, sitting with God on the brink of eternity while being served by those of many colors and ethnicities. God bless them!

Chapter 23

•

Black Tax and White Benefits – Stop Black Tax!

S o, what should we do about God's obvious love of great variety and the fact that no scientific or biblical evidence is to be found for the common view of race? The answer to this question is a simple one but far from being easy to put into practice. We who are White must start getting educated about the world the Black person is living in and then act upon what we are learning, especially as it relates to our relationships in the church. The world is broken and will never be fixed, since it is under Satan's control, but Christ is the head of the church and can fix us if we will allow him to do it. One thing is for sure, he wants us to love our fellow brothers and sisters in his family and to demonstrate that love in every way possible.

Scores if not hundreds of verses could be quoted which show us the ways our love should be expressed in our spiritual family, but here are two. "Carry each other's burdens, and in this way you will fulfill the law of Christ" (Galatians 6:2). "Rejoice with those who rejoice; mourn with those who mourn" (Romans 12:15). I cannot help carry another's burdens without first knowing what they are. I cannot mourn with those who mourn without knowing the source of their grief and its depth. When I was a kid growing up in the Jim Crow days of Louisiana, America was totally controlled by White people. Honestly, it still mostly is. Our Black brothers and sisters (and others of color) have learned to adapt to our world. Most have a very difficult time letting us know what that world is really like to them—unless we start asking.

When I almost died in the hospital, large numbers of people were asking about how I was doing and praying for me. They were asking my wife and other family members how they were feeling. When someone we know has a severe financial crisis, like having their house burn down, we want to know what they are feeling and facing. We want to help. When a fellow disciple loses a loved one, we want to find out how they are feeling and comfort them. We want to feel their pain and help bear their burdens in any way possible. You get the point, right? In many areas of emotional or physical or financial pain, we want to discover what others are experiencing and feeling about those experiences. Why do we not have the same concern for those who live in a world that stereotypes them very negatively in both obvious and subtle ways without even thinking about it?

Back in 2016, I started a blog entitled, "Black Tax and White Benefits," to start trying to help educate my fellow White disciples and to encourage disciples of color to handle their challenges in the racial realm spiritually. The genesis of my efforts traces back to ten days after a tragedy occurred in Dallas on July 7, 2016. Two Black men had recently been killed by White policemen, one in Minnesota and another in Louisiana. A protest march was taking place in Dallas when a heavily armed Black man, Micah Xavier Johnson, opened fire on police officers, killing five and wounding nine other officers and two civilians.

Ten days later, on July 17, I was asked to speak in the Southwest Region of the DFW Church, a Region composed of a half White and half non-White membership and served by a ministry staff of the same racial ratio. Mark Mancini, the leader of the Region, asked me to come and speak to the group on the subject of racism and the Bible. Although I had addressed the subject many times in sermons for decades, it was the first time I had preached an entire sermon on the topic. As others heard about the sermon or listened to a recording of it online, I received requests to preach the same lesson in a number of places, inside and outside Dallas. I began to get educated quickly and deliberately from that point and decided to start my blog soon afterwards.

The term "Black Tax" came from a movie I watched in which a Black woman described it as having to do her job twice as well as a White person to be given the same credit, and her role in the show demonstrated the point quite well. Amazingly, Delta Airlines helped me explain the issue very clearly just prior to starting the blog. Here's a quote from the second post on my blog.

> Two blatant examples took place within days of each other last month (October) involving black female doctors flying on Delta Airlines. Two medical emergencies occurred, prompting flight attendants to ask for help from medically trained passengers. In both cases, the black doctors reportedly tried to answer the call to help, only to be rebuffed by the flight attendants because they couldn't picture black women being doctors.

In a talk with my African American neighbor, she added that the term "Black tax" is also commonly used within the Black community to describe the stresses that Black people feel in most settings, knowing that they are being stereotyped negatively by White people any time they are out in public settings. These stresses are not only real; they are dangerous to the health of Black people. The statistics are undeniable. Being Black in America means that your health and longevity may well be affected. A brief examination of pregnancy complications or heart disease of the Black population makes the point, in addition to other maladies. Black people don't say much about this type of Black tax they are paying because they know they have to fit in or suffer consequences that they are trying hard to avoid.

The term "White Benefits" started off in the title of my blog as "White Privilege," but one of my advisors recommended avoiding that term in the title because of the political environment and reactions to the term. That said, I didn't avoid using the term as a title for one of my blog posts, explaining it like this:

> White privilege is not so much what you have; it is what you don't have—stereotypical treatment of the worst kind. A fairly recent segment of "Dr. Phil" was devoted to showing what White privilege is. He is quite in tune with the topic, as were his panelists. As Michael Burns puts it: "White privilege does not mean that you did not have obstacles and challenges in life; it means that your skin color or culture wasn't one of them." That's the bottom-line issue.

As a White person deeply concerned for the "world" in which my Black brothers and sisters live, I have talked to hundreds of Black people inside and outside the church about their experiences, challenges and feelings. I have read extensively materials about the topic from those who know more than I do about it. I have watched many video podcasts on YouTube and a number of documentaries on TV. When I was developing my podcast series, I asked to meet with one of my Black brothers from my ministry group and gave him the following questions to think about in advance and then to address when we met.

1. As a Black person, what would you like your White friends to know about what hurts you? Please break these down into deep hurts and those less hurtful but still painful. Maybe

number them by depth of pain, starting with the worst to you personally.

2. Second, by prioritizing again, what things would you most like to see change in your White disciple friends? Break this one down into their attitudes and their actions.

3. Those are WPQs (White person questions). Is there a better way to come at this from a Black person's perspective?

4. What do I (Gordon) do that does or could hit a Black person the wrong way. Since I am trying to learn, Black people appreciate that and likely cut me some slack. Those of us who are trying to learn are the ones who shouldn't be given slack. I don't want a free pass. I want to learn.

As it turned out, he didn't address each of the questions. But they stirred his thinking and feelings enough to take advantage of the opportunity to express what was really on his heart. I made sure he did address #4, which was very helpful to me as I continue to learn more about myself. I yet have much to learn despite how much I have already learned. The starting place is the decision to get started, don't you think?

For us White people, we are long past the point of being able to claim innocence through ignorance. It is way past time to face the facts, stop accepting the "spin" given on the topic by White people, especially politically oriented ones, and start obeying God's directions given in verses like I quoted earlier. I'm simply asking you, in the name of Christ, to get involved in caring, learning, conversing and loving. We cannot love in generalities, so let's start showing our love in the specifics—the ones described in this lesson. God bless us all to demonstrate his love to all of our fellow disciples in every realm, the racial one for sure. In his name, let's eradicate every vestige of Black tax in the family of God. Amen! I love you!

Conclusion

Why did God put the writing of this book on my heart? What did he hope to accomplish through it? Those questions cannot be answered with certainty, but I hope that his purposes align closely with mine, and I know what I hope the book did for you. First, that it helped you in your understanding of God and in your relationship with him. Second, it helped you in how you view and value relationships with other people. Third, it helped you deal with health challenges you have and/or your loved ones have or will have. Fourth, it helped you to both cherish life and accept the inevitability of death. Yesterday is history, tomorrow is a mystery, but today is God's gift to us—which is why we call it the present, his present to us all. May you live each of your todays to the full and may the lessons in this book help you to do just that.

In Acts 20:27, Paul said that he had "not hesitated to proclaim to you the whole will of God." That is my calling as well. I have spent the years trying to teach the whole counsel of God, focusing primarily on teaching others how to live. Before I pack it in, I have the responsibility and opportunity to also teach others how to die. Again, some might be thinking, "Gordon, that's morbid!" The dictionary might agree, with this definition: "characterized by or appealing to an abnormal and unhealthy interest in disturbing and unpleasant subjects, especially death and disease." But I most certainly do not agree that these subjects are morbid. They are a part of life. Something will stop our heart and we will leave this realm and journey into the next. None of us are exempt. God is trying to prepare us for life and for death. I am a teacher and I want to be used by God to do my best to help you with both parts. That's not morbid; that's life, life with God.

My fellow teacher and friend, Douglas Jacoby, set up a phone conversation with me just to catch up and see how I was doing during the early stages of my cancer battle. He told me about a book that a man wrote about his life which was in the process of winding to a close through a terminal disease. Doug suggested that if the cancer was going to take me down that road, I could contribute to helping people by following a similar course. I appreciated his suggestion and awoke the next morning with a title in mind, which I wrote into a document designed as a book cover. "Cancer—From Diagnosis to Death." Unless I die suddenly, I may still write that book in some form or another, even if death comes from something besides cancer. We are all going to die, and I want to do it well. I have been blessed to see some do it admirably and inspiringly, examples I want to follow so that others can follow mine.

While I am thankful for my present two-year reprieve from cancer and hope that you have a similar reprieve if you are currently in the midst of a cancer or other serious health challenge, we all must come to peace with our mortality. It most often is going to be a process. If we are fortunate enough to live to an old age, aging itself should usher in the process. In a wonderful book entitled, *An Aging Grace,*[xvii] edited by and written in by Jeanie Shaw and many others, I wrote two chapters. Although that was only about eight years ago, I was not in the best place to write about aging and death. Yet, those were the topics Jeanie assigned me. God has such a sense of humor, as does Jeanie. You should read the book, and I think you will enjoy my two chapters. I am nothing if not candid in them. My title for chapter two of the book was, "Aging Grace,

How Sweet the Sound?" and my title for chapter thirty-four, the final chapter, was, "The Best Is Yet to Be." I needed to write those chapters, for they were a part of my preparation for playing my own end game. What I wrote then I fully believed intellectually but hadn't fully reached the point of accepting it emotionally. I'm there now, thanks to cancer—a part of the bigger picture. I close with a quote from the last section of that final chapter.

> As it is with aging, death is all a matter of perspective—seeing the material world or seeing the spiritual world. Both are real, but the former one just barely so by comparison. It's a nice place to hang out for a few decades, but it's merely a launching pad to the really real world. I'm thankful to have lived on planet earth, but I was here for only one main reason: to get prepared for blastoff to the next. A baby in the womb is comfortable and peaceful, and when they start to make their entrance into a big new world, it is probably very scary. Life in the womb of this earth is sometimes comfortable and peaceful, and the thought of leaving it might still be a bit scary. But let's allow it to be scary in the same way that astronauts must feel as the flames of rocket fuel start pushing them into a world they have heretofore only imagined.

Endnotes

i. Gordon Ferguson, *The Victory of Surrender, Second Edition* (Woburn, MA: Discipleship Publications International, 1999)

ii. Gordon Ferguson, "Eternity's Brink", YouTube, https://www.youtube.com/results?search_query=eternity%27s+Brink

iii. Gordon Ferguson, *Romans: the Heart Set Free* (Billerica, MA: Discipleship Publications International, 2001)

iv. Gordon Ferguson, "I Have Lost My Faith (in Coincidences)", gordonferguson. org, https://gordonferguson.org/i-have-lost-my-faith-in-coincidences/

v. Gordon Ferguson, *My Three Lives: A Story of One Man and Three Movements* (Spring, TX: Illumination Publishers, 2016)

vi. Jim McGuiggan, *The Book of Ezekiel* (Lubbock, TX: Montex Publishing Company, 1979)

vii. Jim McGuiggan, *The Reign of God* (Lubbock, TX: International Biblical Resources, 1979)

viii. Jim McGuiggan, *The God of the Towel* (West Monroe, LA: Howard Publishing Company, 1997)

ix. Jim McGuiggan, *Jesus Hero of Thy Soul* (West Monroe, LA: Howard Publishing Company, 1998)

x. Gordon Ferguson, *Dynamic Leadership* (Spring, TX: Illumination Publishers, 2012)

xi. Gordon Ferguson, "Life's End Game and the Greatest Story Ever Told", gordonferguson.org, https://gordonferguson.org/lifes-end-game-and-the-greatest-story-ever-told/

xii. Gordon Ferguson, *The Power of Spiritual Relationships* (Spring, TX: Illumination Publishers, 2020)

xiii. Gordon Ferguson, God, *Are We Good?* (Spring, TX: Illumination Publishers, 2020)

xiv. Gordon Ferguson, "Why Are Humans Different Colors?", blacktaxandwhitebenefits.com, https://blacktaxandwhitebenefits.com/archives/459

xv. Gordon Ferguson, "Is the Coronavirus COVID-19 a Judgment of God?", gordonferguson.org, https://gordonferguson.org/is-the-coronavirus-covid-19-a-judgment-of-god/

xvi. Gordon Ferguson, "Just What is White Privilege?", blacktaxandwhitebenefits. com, https://blacktaxandwhitebenefits.com/archives/519

xvii. Jeanie Shaw, *An Aging Grace,* (Spring, TX: Illumination Publishers, 2016)

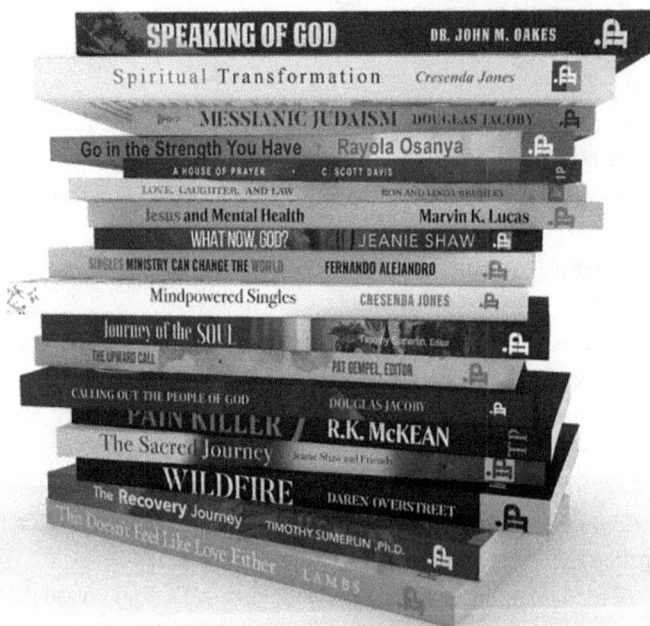

www.ingramcontent.com/pod-product-compliance
Lightning Source LLC
Chambersburg PA
CBHW032058020426
42335CB00011B/394